ISBN-13: 978-1542820011

ISBN-10: 1542820014

Edited by: Randi Chapnik Myers

Coach: Robert Pal

Front Cover Designed by: Liz Wisnieski, borisDezign

Text Design and Layout by: Senka Kubisztal

Printed in the United States of America

THE CONTENTS

THE AUTHOR

Dr. Mayer Hoffer is a psychiatrist who has been in private practice in Toronto, Canada since 1983. A recognized expert in the field of Attention Deficit Hyperactivity Disorder, his clinical work is specialized in the diagnosis and treatment of ADD across the life cycle. Dr. Hoffer holds the following degrees: M.D., Bachelor of Science in Medicine, Fellow of the Royal College of Physicians and Surgeons of Canada, Diplomate of Child Psychiatry, and Diplomate of the American Board of Psychiatry and Neurology. He has also held positions as the medical director of the ADDvance Treatment Centre and the Chief Resident of Child Psychiatry at the Hospital of Sick Children.

PREFACE

Why do you need this book?

Attention Deficit Hyperactivity Disorder aka Attention
Deficit Disorder. These days, the term is so familiar, but how much
do we really know about ADD (I use the terms ADD and ADHD
interchangeably)? We know this for sure: The condition has grown
into a widespread problem and yet, in the field of medicine, ADD is
still woefully misunderstood and ineptly treated. Well, thankfully,
that's all about to change.

We all know many people who are suffering with ADD,
whether diagnosed and undiagnosed. Chances are, you are reading
this book because you have the disorder or you are close to someone
who does, and you are frustrated by the lack of real help available.
You are not alone. The fact is, Attention Deficit Disorder may be the
most common mental health disorder around, with the largest
socioeconomic health impact. So why does it continue to be largely
ignored by the medical and psychiatric profession? And what does
that disregard cost individuals and society as a whole? Simply put, the

2

lack of proper recognition of ADD, particularly in the female and adult populations, has meant that people everywhere are leading frustrated, unfulfilled lives while a disorder that is eminently treatable wreaks havoc on a daily basis.

The good news, for doctors and patients alike, is that there is help for the millions of ADD patients that have been misdiagnosed or have been flying under the radar for so long. In this book, I outline a new conceptual model for the condition, which finally offers safe and effective treatment options that are proven to stop the suffering and help people live their fullest lives.

I wrote this book with the intention of elevating the discourse about Attention Deficit Hyperactivity Disorder beyond the simplistic framework this area of psychiatry and medicine has been mired in for decades. It is not intended to be yet another "ADD handbook" since the market is saturated with those already. Instead, I provide insight into the day-to-day clinical practice of a psychiatrist who has had great success in diagnosing and treating ADD in patients across the life cycle, from preschool to senior citizens.

Whenever a book is written about medical topics that include a discussion of treatment options, a physician needs to be involved. Treatment for any condition should never be posed as a "do-it-yourself" guide and in the case of ADD, there is no doubt that medical/psychiatric supervision is absolutely necessary. That said, I have purposely written this book for both the general public and the medical/psychiatric/psychological professions. My hope is that my experience with ADD will both inform and stimulate discussion, which will in turn propel the profession forward in this area of study and help as many people as possible.

Even though the medical process I describe is what I do in my office every day, the conceptual treatment model and the medication regimens I advocate are revolutionary. In particular, the medication combinations I use to treat patients are not currently accepted as the "norm" of ADD treatment. Though I hope that my methodology will become the "gold standard" of ADD treatment, it is not yet considered standard operating procedure.

The treatment approach that I utilize is intended to and often does achieve a robust therapeutic result, and indeed, a transformative one. And as you'll read, this positive outcome is common. But no single treatment works for every patient. That said, the title of book references the "game-changing" quality of my treatment protocol. For the person with ADD who exhibits both the difficulty of regulating attention and the lifelong quandary of procrastination and poor decision-making, getting both sides of the ADD coin addressed and treated can eventually "change the game" of life.

I have tried to clearly explain the "science component" of this issue in a fashion that even those with no medical background can grasp. I hope that by the end of the book, medical and non-medical readers alike will feel knowledgeable about the workings of the brain's "neurotransmission" in the case of people with Attention Deficit Disorder.

While here, I primarily discuss the presence and treatment of ADD in adults, keep in mind that many of the same principles I describe are applicable to children and teenagers with ADD with some important modifications. My next book will focus on how revolutionary treatment protocol is desperately needed in the field of children and adolescents with Attention Deficit Disorder as well.

A few acknowledgements to those who helped to bring this book to life. Much appreciation goes to my colleague Robert Pal, ADD Coach, for reading through the pages and offering me encouragement along the way. To my secretary Senka Kubisztal for typing my longhand writing and providing me with feedback. To my editor, Randi Chapnik Myers, who cleaned up the text and taught me about the wonders of Google Docs. And finally, to my wife Fern, whom I love so much, for her support during the birthing process of this manuscript.

CHAPTER 1

<u>Really? That's the best you can do?</u>

When I give talks about Attention Deficit Disorder (ADD) to groups of physicians, I describe the "classic case" of ADD as the female university student who shows up at the University Health and Counselling Services in November of her first semester. I do so because most doctors today still view ADD as a male illness only. Clever and resourceful enough to achieve high credit scores in her final two years of high school, the young woman gained admission to her university of choice. She has a lovely personality, is articulate, and presents herself very well. She has come from a supportive home where her mother nudged her to complete homework and from a supportive school environment where kindly teachers gave regular reminders of assignment due dates as they neared. A solid student by all accounts, she kicked off the university academic term in September with high hopes and expectations of success.

But things have not worked out as expected. The young lady is floundering in her new environment. She can't figure out how her peers seem to be able to handle this new life so much more easily—figuring out where to get groceries and when to get laundry done, organizing to get to class on time, prioritize readings, get assignments completed and turned in, and the list goes on. She starts to feel like everyone around her is part of a club of "regular effective people" while she sits on the outside. In my practice, I often use the expression that the patient feels that he or she was not in the lineup when the "royal jelly" was being handed out.

Upset by her lack of effectiveness and capacity, the young woman walks into the consultation room. The psychiatrist at the university clinic greets her and asks what brings her to the appointment.

"I'm not doing well," she replies. "I can't seem to organize myself properly. I'm forever leaving things to the last minute even when I know I shouldn't be procrastinating. I've fallen behind and I'm fearful that I'm not going to pass my end-of-term examination. I have no idea what I'm going to tell my parents when I go home for Christmas break."

The learned psychiatrist, often with two or three hyphens bolstering his last name, immediately probes with the classic question: "How do you *feel* about that?"

"Not too good," the young lady responds.

"So how long have you been depressed for?" the doctor asks.

What has just happened here? If you are wondering what I am referring to, then join the crowd. It seems like such a straightforward interaction, doesn't it? But it's not. And for the young lady, this conversation has the potential to be life altering and devastating. Why is that? And why am I making such a big deal out of it?

This student—and countless others like her who are suffering from Attention Deficit Disorder all over the world—has presented herself at the University Health Services at a critical juncture in her young life and stated, "I am not *doing* well." Doing. What she is describing here is a *function* problem, not an illness problem. However, what the psychiatrist has done, in the initial seconds of this important interaction, is made an automatic illness diagnosis. Specifically, he has slid the young woman's diagnostic assessment into the psychiatrist's comfort zone, which is a feeling category, labelled depression or anxiety, or depression/anxiety, or if he is very sophisticated, anxiety/depression.

This tendency to diagnose function problems as illness is way too common in psychiatry. I make the joke when I give talks about Attention Deficit Disorder that I could be stumbling down drunk on a bad day and I can still diagnose and treat depression and anxiety.

What then ensues? The young lady may be offered a few follow-up counselling sessions. More often than not, given the constraints of availability of resources and time, she will be given a prescription for a serotonin-related antidepressant (aka the SSRI family, which includes Prozac, Celexa, Cipralex, Zoloft, etc.). Seen in follow up three weeks later, the psychiatrist returns to the same line of questioning: "And how are you *feeling* now?"

"Not as anxious as I was," she replies.

The psychiatrist, so pleased with his clinical acumen, practically contorts his body to reach over and pat his own back for being such a skilled and helpful doctor.

But what he fails to do is ask the important function question: "And how are you *doing?*" If he did follow up with function, he would hear some variation on the following: "I guess I'm not cut out for university; I thought I was smart enough but I'm not. I'm still not getting my assignments handed in, I haven't caught up on my readings; I'm way behind on my studying. I still can't get started on things; I'm so disorganized. I'm not planning to come back to school after Christmas—there's no point. I'm going to look for a job somewhere." In other words, the patient's problem persists.

Sadly for too many people who live with ADD, this story is not rare. In fact, it is so common that I wouldn't be surprised if you have already identified yourself in the description of what has taken place.

What happens next? This same university coed goes out into the world. Her confidence has been dealt a crippling blow. She is now at greater risk for being unable to maintain employment and stay in a successful committed relationship, and she is more likely to engage in drug and alcohol abuse. This is also the patient who is seen 10, 20 and 30 years later in the psychiatrist or psychologist or psychotherapist's office—always with the same presentation. She is nice, lacking in confidence, smart but underachieved to the level of her intellect, always feeling flustered and overwhelmed, particularly if she has to multi-task, with a string of failed trials of psychotherapy, counseling, antidepressants and anti-anxiety medications behind her. Worst of all, she always leaves with the same diagnosis: depression/anxiety/depression/anxiety.

And here is the rub. That desultory outcome is avoidable. So much so that, on assessing a patient with this all too common story, I will tell the young lady that her presentation is a walk in the park for me to treat. I tell her she should expect a big and robust response to treatment; that if she only sees some little mincing miserable response then the treatment needs to change. I tell her that I will be shocked if I don't do a good job for her. I explain that it would be to my advantage to tell her exactly the opposite, that her presentation is very complex and challenging and that it will take all of my vast clinical expertise to see if I can achieve any improvement at all, but that's not the truth. So either I am a big talker or when it comes to ADD patients, I have a clue, as I've been here many, many times before.

To offer ADD patients false hope, albeit in some well-intended but misguided way, would be cruel and misleading. And the last time I checked, nobody would describe me that way. I tell my patient that I am not trying to plant the seed of hopeful expectation with the intention of playing on her desperate desire to do better. On the contrary, because what I do is results-oriented, I encourage patients to remain skeptical until they see the result. What is most important, I explain, is that they remain accurate in their reporting back to me as I will work hard to be accurate with them; if the patient only tells me what they think I want to hear, the exercise will prove to be a waste of our time, for both of us.

And finally I tell my patient, while dressed in my T-shirt and jeans, that nobody comes to see me because I'm such a snappy dresser.

In this book, I will outline how I understand ADD, how I conceptualize it, the treatment model that I have constructed that helps guide treatment decisions, and the treatment protocol I use to correct the ongoing functional challenges that hinder adult ADD patients in their daily lives. My hope is that the real-life case studies here will elevate and sharpen the tired old discourse about Attention Deficit Disorder so that it can be properly treated everywhere for patients seeking help. And if, along the way, you get the impression that the author thinks he's smarter than everyone else, I don't. But what is clear is that I do seem to achieve way better results in my patients than most. That outcome needs to be shared widely and broadly or else millions of people, generations upon generations, will never get the chance to live the life that they are, in fact, fully capable of living.

But first, I will review how we—as psychiatrists and physicians as well as the general public—ended up in the diagnostic and treatment quagmire we find ourselves in currently with respect to Attention Deficit Disorder.

CHAPTER 2

Why is ADD so misunderstood?

The training of a medical student is typically four years in duration and there is lots to learn in that time. The first year is spent digesting a huge amount of basic material—anatomy, physiology, pathology, and the list goes on. The learning of basic science continues into second year, where there is also an exciting introduction to some patient contact. The third and fourth years are largely hospital and clinic-based as the imparting of clinical knowledge proceeds. Fourth year ends with final examinations followed by a hospital-based internship of one to two years, leading to one becoming a general practitioner (GP) or family doctor (FD).

In all of these years of training, the time that a student spends in a psychiatric rotation generally amounts to one to two months in total. During that brief stint, the topic of Attention Deficit Disorder will have been discussed during one lecture, maybe. And yet, ironically, most GPs and FDs who may have found psychiatry "boring and irrelevant" while in school are the first to confide that mental health issues now represent one-third to one-half of their daily workload and they wish they were better trained to deal with it.

After a few years of practicing medicine or immediately after completing the internship, a graduate physician can apply to and, if accepted, enter a three- to four-year residency program to study psychiatry. Currently, a training psychiatrist studies general adult psychiatry, with the option to "specialize" in child and adolescent psychiatry. Here again, in the process of becoming a general adult psychiatrist, the sum total of teaching about ADD is limited to one, or at best two, lectures with some clinical discussion depending on what cases are seen.

That's the good news. The bad news is that what little is taught about Attention Deficit Disorder is frequently outdated and misleading crap. Perhaps most alarming, right from the inception, ADD is improperly positioned. Why am I saying so?

The major psychiatric bible, the Diagnostic and Statistical Manual, Fifth Edition (the DSM-5), which can be found online, outlines the clinical description of Attention Deficit Hyperactivity Disorder (usually referred to as Attention Deficit Disorder or ADD). The name of the condition implies that the patient should have a problem paying attention to things that matter and further, should be fidgety and hyperactive. Though the updated diagnostic criteria allow for a "predominantly inattentive presentation" or a "predominantly hyperactive/impulsive presentation", in broad clinical practice, this distinction is not made. In fact, to this day, if the patient does not appear hyperactive—with what I refer to as the "Mexican jumping bean" appearance—then the diagnosis is not even entertained.

As a result, the majority of ADD patients never receive the proper diagnosis or treatment. In particular, female patients, who are much less likely to demonstrate hyperactivity at all, fail to get properly diagnosed and have to find a way to function in life without understanding what is hindering them.

When I lecture to physicians, I often talk about the "ADD Iceberg". Like an iceberg, where the largest part resides below the waterline, the vast majority of ADD patients are not overtly physically hyperactive. This point is crucial to understand. The fact is, I can speak extemporaneously without notes for two hours about ADD and never mention the word hyperactivity once.

The other misleading aspect of the diagnosis is the obvious emphasis on "attention". Even patients with severe cases of ADD are capable of paying attention if they are very keen on a particular area of interest or when it comes to things they find entertaining. Often they can "hyper focus" and spend hours "locked in" to some activity, such as video games, for instance. However, that hyper focus is not what "attention" references in this context. Rather, it is about being able to maintain and sustain attention for longer periods of time over the course of a day on things one is interested in as well as on things that may bore them to tears (think school).

Now here comes the kicker. In many ADD patients, like the "classic" case I referenced in the preceding chapter, it is neither the attention nor the hyperactivity that is most prominent. Of course, there is a history of weakness in the area of regulating attention but it is in fact in the area of decision making—or executive function—that most people with ADD struggle. These executive functions can be addressed by analyzing the answers to the following questions:

- Are you aware of how you come across to others?
- Can you find, and hit, your own pause button on your own personal "VCR" control so that when faced with a decision, rather than blurting something out or unwisely ignoring it, you can pause, think things through, weigh consequences, and then come to a decision all within microseconds?
- Are you sensitive to other people's perceptions of you?
- Can you be a team player when necessary?
- Can you be flexible and have a sense of humour, particularly under stress?
- Under stress, can you manage and maintain a regular mood?
- Can you pick up on social cues and social nuance?
- Can you time manage properly?
- Can you prioritize properly?
- Can you initiate tasks and then "start, continue, complete"?
- Can you stay motivated, even in the face of frustration?
- Can you avoid procrastinating to your own detriment?

If you work in the field of mental health, think now of how much more completely the preceding list describes patients with ADD. If you are someone who has been frustrated for so long, wondering why the hell you can't get your life on track, and can now see how these questions resonate with your life circumstance, then you are miles ahead of most of the medical/psychological/psychiatry professionals that you have called upon for help. Chances are that those professionals, if they consider ADD at all, are still stuck in that "Attention/Hyperactivity" box along with the rest of the medical community.

What other features of Attention Deficit Disorder lend themselves so readily to misunderstanding? To this day, ADD is thought of as predominantly a "boy's illness". When I was training in psychiatry many decades ago, the male to female ratio for Attention Deficit Disorder was thought to be four boys to one girl—and at that time, adult ADD was felt not to exist. As time passed and the profession became more aware of the condition, the ratio dropped but was still high: 2.5 - 3 male cases to each female case.

So why point to the "classic ADD case" as being a young woman? Because in my opinion there is no gender disparity in Attention Deficit Disorder, whatsoever. There is no "Y chromosome" involvement in ADD and as a result, there are as many female cases as there are male ones. Moreover, the "classic case" highlights three important starting points in any discussion of ADD:

1. Women are just as likely as men to have the condition.
2. ADD is often missed in adulthood.
3. The presence of hyperactivity is not necessary to consider the diagnosis of ADD.

There are other obstacles to understanding ADD with greater clarity as well. According to the DSM-5 criteria, to formally make the diagnosis, "several" of the ADD symptoms must have been present in a patient prior to the age of 12. Although usually, these childhood antecedents can be elicited in a carefully taken history, that "evidence" is not always available. In particular, adult patients may not have parents to provide collateral history, psychological tests and school report cards may be unavailable, and other potential collateral sources may not be pursued due to privacy and confidentiality concerns. Moreover, and this is key to the conceptual understanding of the *functional* nature of the disorder—as opposed to the misperception of ADD as an illness—a very significant number of patients with ADD did not have symptoms in childhood.

If you are starting to think that I am trying to go out of my way to be controversial and take the position of lone wolf/maverick rebel, I can assure you that I am not. What I am trying to convey is an accurate picture of the ADD that I have observed day in and day out over the course of more than three decades of clinical practice. Permit me to explain.

The vast majority of people with Attention Deficit Disorder are smart. They are also almost universally underachieved to the level of their intellect. The fact that they haven't done well in school or have experienced frequent career disappointments, which negatively impact their self esteem and leave them feeling unsuccessful, does not make them any less intelligent. In fact, many people with ADD are so smart that the early years of school offer little or no challenge to their performance capacity. Either they can pay "enough attention to get it" or, as ADD people always end up doing, they develop successful (initially, at least) in-the-moment compensatory strategies to enable them to succeed. They cut corners, they wait until the night before work is due and then perform under pressure, they find friends who take good notes in class, and sometimes, they cheat. Functionally, they adapt as they need to, using a type of survival strategy.

For some, the strategy falls apart early, in elementary school or even earlier. A smaller cohort can sail through high school and perhaps even undergraduate college and university. The largest single factor in the breaking point is often when the level of the intellect and the effectiveness of the compensations can't outweigh the degree of difficulty and complexity of the tasks required. In other words, the functional capacity is no longer able to meet the demands and challenges of one's life. It is not that you have "developed" ADD in your 20's or 30's; it is that your ability to adequately cope is no longer effective. You are, as I refer to this breaking point, "fraying at the seams".

There are many other points of misperception, misunderstanding and reasons for continued willful ignorance pertaining to ADD. Some will be addressed in subsequent chapters. To keep each chapter brief and easily digestible, I will limit myself to just one more difficulty here.

As mentioned earlier, psychiatrists train to be adult psychiatrists and then they can opt for specialized training in child and adolescent psychiatry. (This order of education is unlikely to ever change despite the obvious argument that it makes more sense to reverse it on the "as the twig is bent, so grows the tree" basis.) In child psychiatry, which most adult psychiatrists are unfamiliar with, the overriding principle, nay bias, has always been to use medication only "as a last resort". There are many reasons for this restraint, including a certain obvious common sense to that principle, the current primacy of political correctness and antipathy to non-organic "chemical" treatment like prescribed medications, a general reluctance to prescribe stimulants to children, as well as the fear of being seen as a "pill pusher" and running into medical-legal concerns while rendering yourself vulnerable to criticism from medical regulatory boards.

Early on, treating Attention Deficit Disorder in children ended up being an area where "the optics suck". Prescribing medication to children for problems that many of my psychiatry colleagues don't acknowledge and "don't believe in" (almost as a matter of religious principle) was for many years a lonely and unpopular choice. Even to consider just one medication treatment was a huge hill to climb for many doctors—as well as for many parents of young ADD patients.

There then came a time when the wind started to shift, and society as a whole began to accept that a single medication might be helpful for ADD patients. At that time of change, academic doctors proudly and self-righteously pronounced at medical meetings that a single pharmaceutical agent was now the gold standard for ADD treatment.

Understand as I am writing this that my target audience for this book is both the general public and the medical/psychological/psychiatric profession. Now understand that there is almost no other area of medicine, including psychiatry, that has treated large category illness with just a single pharmaceutical agent the same way for 40 years and counting. Think asthma, high blood pressure, arthritis, depression. If a specialist were to stand up and declare that a single treatment for any of those illnesses is the gold standard and we should almost never consider a second or third contemporaneously prescribed medication treatment, they would be laughed out of the room. The idea would be preposterous. Except when it comes to ADD.

Why? Because the optics suck. The evil crazed fuzzy haired mad scientist/shrink shoveling evil toxins down the throats of pure children or misguided vulnerable adults is not the warm and fuzzy picture we want to see. That's why it matters so much that we always look beyond the optics, especially when it comes to Attention Deficit Disorder.

CHAPTER 3

Why does ADD matter so much?

It is generally recognized that today, ADD is present in approximately 10% of children and teenagers—and that is definitely a modest approximation. Approximately 10 years ago, the American Society of Pediatrics published a paper that suggested the number to be as high as 16%.

In the late 70s, when I was training to become a psychiatrist, we were taught that Attention Deficit Disorder was not a particularly big deal and in any case, most children would "outgrow" it by the time they started adolescence. In fact, to validate the prevailing notion of that time, we were taught that, should a child require psychostimulant medication (generally Ritalin back then) at all, and only then as a "last resort", we should be ever vigilant to monitor the young lad (girls were rarely diagnosed) as he entered his teen years for the "adolescent switch". This was the golden moment when, under the pressure of hormonally-driven neurophysiological development, the child's immature brain would have finally evolved to the point where the child would announce, "Mama, Papa, I have noticed in the past few days that my medication, which used to help me focus and concentrate, is now causing me to be very inattentive and easily agitated and overactive." At that moment, the child would have "turned on the switch" and would formally and conclusively be "over" his ADD.

Not only was this trajectory inaccurate—the "adolescent switch" is almost never seen—but it also served to propagate the belief that an ADD diagnosis didn't really matter all that much. After all, you were going to outgrow it anyway.

More than 30 years ago, back when ADD was still not widely recognized, a U.S. study examined the prevalence of ADD symptomatology in new patients presenting to the hospital-based outpatient child psychiatric department for any reason. At that time, more than 50% of the patients presenting had what appeared to be ADD symptoms. Not surprisingly, most of those patients were not being seen for a primary diagnosis of ADD but rather were being treated for other diagnostic categories, including behaviour disorder, depression, anxiety, delinquency, and others. Even more alarming, that number is almost certainly an under-representation of the total number of ADD patients, not only because of the era but also because non-hyperactive children were not identified as ADD at all.

Return to the 10% number, the estimate of children who have Attention Deficit Disorder today. What is the current thinking about how many ADD children and teenagers continue to show significant diagnosable ADD symptoms into adulthood? The generally accepted figure is 60%. In other words, 10 out of every 100 children have ADD and 6 of those 10 children will carry their symptoms into adulthood.

Now let's return to the figure I quoted previously where 50% or more in the pediatric population were seeking psychiatric help with ADD as part of the picture. Do you really think that these individuals, with poor decision-making and deficient impulse control, low achievement at school, who now find themselves sliding down the socioeconomic ladder, might not also be overrepresented in the offices and clinics of adult psychiatrists? Shockingly, though, most of my adult psychiatric colleagues still will not diagnose Attention Deficit Disorder and as a result, they do not treat it either. Sounds a bit crazy, doesn't it?

So what are the numbers when it comes to Adult ADD? Consider the following. If you have ADD (untreated, usually undiagnosed), you are 5-6 times as likely to not finish high school, twice as likely to be involved in a serious car accident, twice as likely to have obesity, 3-4 times as likely to be a habitual smoker, 3 times as likely to be divorced and 4 times as likely to have a psychiatric hospitalization. You are 3-4 times as likely to be incarcerated and 3-4 times as likely to develop a substance abuse (drugs and/or alcohol) disorder. From a socioeconomic perspective, the adult with ADD will have an annual salary 60% of his or her matched age cohort, lower occupational levels, and poorer work performance.

These numbers represent a severe toll on society—job loss,

family dissolution, motor vehicle deaths and injuries, incarcerations—that dwarfs the socioeconomic cost of other psychiatric disorders. And still, there has been very little response by the profession.

Still not convinced? Let me break down just one of those categories: substance abuse. Anyone who has struggled personally with addictions, or has watched a family member fall into the sinister world of alcoholism and/or drug addiction, knows well the devastation associated with it. When I lecture to physicians, I often quote that by the age of 28 (when a person has had some time to be an adult), an undiagnosed and untreated individual with ADD is 4–5 times more likely to develop a substance abuse disorder. The generally accepted figure for lifetime risk of drugs and/or alcohol addiction is 9% of the total population. Now, if 6% of the population has ADD, then it follows that approximately 30–40% of people with substance abuse problems also have ADD.

Now here is where the scenario gets worse. I often say that treating ADD gives a person a chance to function at a much more capable and successful level, which can be protective against developing drug and alcohol abuse habits. The why is obvious. If your ADD is treated, you are more capable of success; you are more confident; your self esteem is higher; you are less likely to feel marginalized; you are less likely to hang out with other marginalized people looking for alternative "ways out" like drugs and alcohol.

However, if you have fallen into a bad drug/alcohol pattern, and you determine that you need to straighten out and you take the important, courageous step to seek psychological/psychiatric help, and you even suspect you have ADD, guess what doesn't happen? That's right. You won't get the proper diagnosis or treatment. Instead, you'll be told that you are at too great a risk for abusing your ADD medications or "diverting them" by selling them to your druggie friends. In other words, the very issue that may have "greased the skids" for you to fall into the nether world of drugs and alcohol abuse, and the very issue that could help bring you out of it, will not be considered.

There is a similar problem occurring in today's jail systems. Anyone involved in the correctional system is very aware of the high prevalence of Attention Deficit Disorder among the inmate population. Because ADD people are bad eggs? No, because if you are a young person who has a tendency to be impulsive, you lack that pause button to be able to stop, think things through, weigh the consequences, and you can't seem to keep a job. So when a buddy says, "Hey, let's do this!" about a bad idea, you are much more likely to say yes than no.

It is no surprise that one of the greatest challenges in the correctional system is the depressing frequency with which people end up repeating patterns of behaviour that result in repeat incarcerations. The term used to describe this phenomenon is recidivism. There is a whole section of criminology and behavioural psychology devoted to the study of trying to reduce the rate of recidivism, which, despite huge efforts and vast sums of money expended, remains stubbornly high.

Now it would be egregious of me to blithely assert that I

know the most important singular ingredient missing in the treatment recipe of incarcerated individuals. Criminal behaviour is tremendously complex and multifactorial. But if you have ADD, and you are in jail, and you are impulsive, and you are released into the community and nothing is done to address the central issue that led you to jail in the first place, then best of luck. Recognizing, treating and maintaining treatment for ADD is one of the singular most impactful variables that would reduce repetitive criminal behaviour. And nobody says boo about it.

At the same time as Attention Deficit Disorder is being overlooked in a huge component of the general population, there is a tendency within psychiatry to over-diagnose depression and anxiety. In particular, let's address a very challenging area of psychiatric clinical practice in the field of mood disorders: Treatment Resistant Depression (TRD).

There is a disproportionately high percentage of clinical work done by treating psychiatric clinicians to address TRD. It even comes with its own definition—cases of Major Depressive Disorder that do not respond adequately to appropriate courses of at least two antidepressants from two separate antidepressant categories. In sharp contrast to how ADD is treated, it is not unusual for a mood disorders expert, particularly one with clinical expertise in psychopharmacology, to prescribe two or three antidepressants at the same time while also using two or three other augmenting medication treatment modalities—an atypical antipsychotic, a mood stabilizer, an anti-seizure medication, and a soupcon of anti-anxiety pills on an as-needed basis.

For many decades now, all of the efforts to treat depression were aimed at the all-important mood component, the "how are you feeling?" aspect. At the same time, the "thinking" or "cognitive" piece of the puzzle was ignored. The clinical case example I use to convey the importance of stepping "out of the box" to consider a more comprehensive understanding of depression is that of the patient referred by the family doctor for treatment of depression related to work stress. The referring physician has already initiated short-term disability leave from work as well as antidepressant treatment, which the patient has partially responded to.

Next, the psychiatric specialist, utilizing great clinical acumen, adjusts or changes the antidepressant, schedules a series of sessions for supportive psychotherapy or Cognitive Behaviour Therapy (CBT), and considers augmentation strategies to the psychopharmacologic regimen, typically adding in a low dose atypical antipsychotic to reduce anxiety and improve mood. The treatment works. The patient's mood improves and anxiety lessens. Praise is heaped.

Now, what will happen to this patient over the course of the next 2-3 months? Let's say she returns to work, usually on a graduated return-to-work schedule. She continues to have follow-up monitoring and support from her family doctor and/or the psychiatrist. As her work schedule becomes more full-time, and the reasonable expectations of the workplace increase in a commensurate fashion, the patient starts to feel flustered at not being able to keep up with the pace of the work flow.

As the patient falls further and further behind, she repeats that she feels she is "floundering" and feels increasingly desperate because of it (though not necessarily more depressed). At this point, adjustments are made to her antidepressant medication regimen. Fingers are nervously crossed.

As the situation deteriorates, still with all the clinical spotlight firmly trained on the "how are you feeling?" component (mood and anxiety), one of two things occur. The patient either requests a return to short-term disability status (which frequently would eventuate into long-term disability) to avoid getting fired. Or the patient gets fired. And diagnostically? All the paperwork would lament the sticky intransigence of tough-to-treat depression aka TRD.

Really? Really? That's the best we can do?

I am a full-time clinician. I see patients all day, day in and day out. I am not a researcher. But I have steadfastly been talking about the importance of "thinking" (cognition is the term psychiatrists and psychologists use) and "functioning" in the assessment and treatment of depressed patients for decades. Some of my colleagues have listened but many have turned a deaf ear with something along the lines of "There goes Hoffer, blathering away about ADD again." But whether or not you are a believer, there is another important question to ask besides how are you feeling? These follow-up questions relate to function and they are crucial: How are you functioning? How are you doing? Are you able to sustain your attention on your work, even when it is repetitive and dull? Asking these questions is really not so hard. But they are really, really important.

For many years now, I have maintained that as much as 30-40% of Treatment Resistant Depression is in fact undiagnosed and untreated Attention Deficit Disorder. I believe that if you address the thinking/doing/functioning aspect of patients who are fearful all day long that they aren't one of the "regular effective people" or that if anyone "looks behind the veil they will see that there is nothing there", everything will change for them. Many of these patients will finally get a chance to gain traction in their life.

A colleague of mine, a specialist in mood and anxiety disorders, Dr. Martin Katzman, is a superb clinician, teacher and researcher. A few years ago, the "penny dropped" and he started to recognize the same pattern of ADD symptoms in many of his mood disorder patients. Today, he is engaged in a research study examining this very phenomenon. He too has become highly frustrated with the obstinate reluctance of our psychiatric colleagues to recognize and address this problem and the failure to view it from another angle.

Dr. Katzman also possesses a wicked wit. He now refers to TRD as DRT, meaning "Doctors Refusing to Treat"—the accompanying underlying ADD, that is.

CHAPTER 4

Why won't (or can't) doctors treat ADD?

In Chapter 3, I touched on the lack of training and clinical exposure that predisposes doctors to maintain their state of "not-knowing-enough-about-this-ADD-stuff" and pointed out the unfortunate DRT phenomena (Doctors Refusing to Treat). What else has led to the dramatic reluctance to acknowledge, address and treat Attention Deficit Disorder in adults? And why am I so intent on discovering an important breakthrough that will advance the understanding of ADD in the medical field?

I grew up in Winnipeg, Manitoba. My hometown is the Canadian exemplar of Midwestern pragmatism, something like the "show-me state" of Missouri. Winnipeg is very much an "I'll believe it when I see it" sort of place. It is also very cold. The old joke is that in Winnipeg we had two seasons—nine months of winter and three months of poor skating. I attended school there and enrolled in pre-med in the Faculty of Science of the University of Manitoba. Back then, going away to university was a dream reserved for wealthy fancy people only.

I excelled at my studies, partly I maintain because it was too cold to do anything but study. I gained early acceptance to medical school and ploughed through four years of medical training. As graduation approached in 1978, I was eager to leave home to expand my horizons. In Canada, the "Big Apple" is Toronto and, like New York City in the U.S., it draws many young people eager to congregate in a larger, more cosmopolitan milieu than the same-old, same-old small town one grew up in. I completed my one-year internship and had to decide whether to start medical practice as a family doctor or continue training to become a specialist.

During my training, I was drawn to two areas of medicine: surgery and psychiatry. Though they seem to be totally divergent, I was drawn to both. Surgery appealed to the part of my personality that likes to be a "doer", to be active. The image of the dynamic handsome surgeon, a la the swashbuckling pirate, who would step into a situation and get things done instead of just talking about it, was very attractive indeed.

The other was psychiatry. It wasn't mental illness per se that drew me but I was fascinated by what makes people tick. And it seemed, at the time, that psychiatry was a more thought provoking and intellectually sophisticated part of the medical world. Coming from my hometown, anything that might help me appear more worldly scored points with me. And, truth be told, except for the absence of a beard that I could thoughtfully stroke, I looked more like a junior egghead Einstein than a soap opera star surgeon. So psychiatry it was, perhaps in spite of the medical joke that surgeons knew nothing but did everything while psychiatrists knew nothing and did nothing.

Next, I embarked on a 4-year residency (training) program to become a psychiatrist. During that time, I decided, based on my lifelong desire to help children, to subspecialize in child and adolescent psychiatry. When I graduated in June 1983, after an interminably long and arduous period of post-secondary education, I was ready to break away from university/school/hospital/bureaucracy settings and open my own psychiatry office, develop a practice, and see patients. And be sophisticated.

When I opened my child and adolescent psychiatry practice, my intention was to become an omniscient, wise, and intellectually deep practitioner. Psychoanalysis and its cousin, psychoanalytically-based psychotherapy, held great sway in the field of that era in Toronto and New York and I had every intention of using my vast intellect (after all, I was smart) and the benevolent milk of kindness coursing through my veins (after all, I was a "mensch") to help troubled children and teenagers. My plan was to accomplish all this through the sheer force of my personhood—my personality and my wisdom. Back then, I'm not even sure that I owned a prescription pad. Or if I did, I would hardly ever use it. Using "pills" was seen as an admission that the primary instrument of your main treatment modality, the force of one's will, was feeble and deficient.

And so I began my career as a child psychiatrist. Starting out in practice was so enjoyable. I was proud that my office was packed from the first day. Of course, I attributed my busy-ness to the lustre of my burgeoning reputation rather than the shortage of child psychiatrists and the resounding success of mailed announcement cards to all the doctors in town. I was busy seeing lots and lots of patients.

Any doctor, and in particular any specialist, will tell you that there is always a huge amount to learn in the practice of medicine and that in the first few years, there is a steep learning curve. There is so much one doesn't know, or doesn't have a granular grip on, that it is imperative that a physician is open to learning throughout his or her career. The image of the pompous arrogant "I'm-the-Doctor!" type of physician is a setup for disaster. We all have to be humble and be willing to question ourselves and others along this lifelong learning process.

Unfortunately, too many doctors feel a great deal of pressure to appear as if they know everything about everything. In particular, my psychiatric colleagues can get very prickly and combative when they are confronted by patients asking them questions about Attention Deficit Disorder. Most of them don't know too much about the area and are nervous about their lack of knowledge and familiarity. And in psychiatry, it is fairly easy for a clinician to divert any discussion away from ADD, using the "bullshit baffles brains" approach. I am forever dumbstruck by the number of new patients who tell me how many times they have approached doctors with their worries of ADD only to be told that "it's not important" or "it doesn't exist" or "we'll look at that after I treat your depression/anxiety/personality disorder" or "there are much deeper issues to look at here".

But I'm getting ahead of myself. I was busy, really busy. I was working hard at what I considered to be my craft. I was so pleased and excited when I would help a young patient and they and their family would let me know what a good/great doctor I was. I was pretty proud of myself. Most of the time, that is.

If you are a good doctor, a really good doctor, you don't linger at the end of the workday on your triumphs and successes. What you remember, what starts to bug you, what rankles you as you lie awake at night, are the patients you are not successful in helping. There is the kid who is just not getting better. Who is not doing well at school. Who doesn't have friends or can't seem to keep new ones around. Then there's the mother with the baleful look on her face telling you that her child has been suspended again or has been asked to look for a new school. Or the teen who seems smart but doesn't hand in assignments—ever—and is dropping out of school.

As I got busier and busier, seeing more and more patients, something started to hammer me over the head time and again. It was this growing group of children and teenagers who looked like they had this attentional challenge along with a lot of impulsivity that seemed more and more likely to be that "attention deficit" story that wasn't supposed to be so prevalent. Moreover, the kids who had it were stubbornly not outgrowing it when they were supposed to. And that wasn't all. I was a supposedly smart child psychiatry specialist and I didn't know very much about what was going on here. Even if I had wanted to, I couldn't ignore this phenomenon because the kids I was treating weren't getting better. And you have to know how bugged I was by that.

So I started to learn as much I could about Attention Deficit Disorder. I read stuff. I read more and more. I conferred with my colleagues in the field of psychology. I dug out my prescription pads.

Remember, too, the era. Even more than now, giving pills to kids was frowned upon. Media reports, particularly those emanating from California, came splashed with sensational headlines such as *Stimulants caused kid to kill grandparents*. Sanctimonious physicians, from the protected sinecures of their lofty academic appointments, railed against the use of psychostimulants as "giving speed to kids." I can't count how many times I watched colleagues, who had to be seeing the same type of patients I was seeing and experiencing the same type of miserable failure that I was experiencing, climb over each other to be first to the microphone to proclaim that they "prefer to emphasize skills, not pills" for their patients—always to earnest applause and nods from the crowd.

As an aside, it was only many years later that the source of almost all of those fabricated ADD horror stories was revealed. It was a media division within the Church of Scientology, which was part of a massive effort to attract followers as part of its marketing efforts to compete for psychotherapy/help seeking dollars.

It was in this milieu that I worked to improve my ability to diagnose and treat Attention Deficit Disorder. Reluctantly, I started to use the psychostimulants that were available at that time, Ritalin (generic name methylphenidate) and Dexedrine. When I would see a young child or teen with a clear history of having difficulty paying attention along with a history of being fidgety and hyperactive, I would initiate a trial of one of the short-acting stimulants, which lasted four hours, as long-acting stimulants were not yet available. The starting dose was low, to be taken immediately after breakfast. A few days later, I would start the second dose immediately after lunch. I would then "tailor" the dose upwards, trying to balance the *negative side effects* (decreased appetite, delayed sleep onset, dry mouth, mild headache, and the possibility of unwanted eye twitches or tics) with the *positive effects* (improved ability to sustain attention for longer, being less distractible, being able to sit at one's desk for longer). Older children and teenagers frequently required an after school dose as well to assist with homework.

Despite my initial trepidations—would the young child grow a third eye in the middle of his forehead? — I found myself relieved and delighted with how relatively easy the process was at first. Most of my young patients responded very well. Side effects (particularly diminished appetite and delayed sleep onset) generally ameliorated within 2-4 weeks. Many children were delighted to be able to maintain their focus and concentration for longer periods. They experienced more success academically than they ever had before. Many were able to make and keep friends, often for the first time.

There were challenges, too, of course. Some children experienced a "crash" or a "rebound" of exaggerated emotionality and hyperactivity as the final short-acting dose wore off at the end of the last dosing. A number of patients had troubling experiences with motor tics (eye twitches, shoulder shrugs, rubbing the corners of their mouth until they were red).

But, for the most part, I thought myself pretty swish. I was starting to help a lot of kids who were thought of as hopeless cases—lazy/crazy/stupid/bad—and I was getting a result. I felt I was onto something. At the very least, I was developing, if not expertise, at least some familiarity with this challenging situation.

But the more patients I treated, and the better I got at understanding this ADD thing, the more incomplete the results seemed. Though I was certainly helping a large number of patients, and even enabling a dramatic transformation in some cases, I started to notice a striking pattern developing. After a few weeks (or a couple of months for patients with an initial "honeymoon period" of early success with dramatically improved focus and concentration), two thirds or more of patients would report that, although they were still clearly able to focus and sustain their concentration for longer, they weren't doing all that much better.

More specifically, the preeminent theme of near unanimous weakness that my ADD patients were noting was that of procrastination/motivation difficulties. These patients would come back and report: "Look Dr. Hoffer, I've always had trouble paying attention for longer periods of time, particularly if I wasn't interested in the subject I was learning about. And then I wouldn't do my homework because I knew I wouldn't be able to stick at it long enough anyway. But then when my treatment started to work really well and I could pay way better attention, I expected that my trouble getting down to my homework would completely fade. But how crazy is this? I can pay attention really well now but I'm still procrastinating. How nuts is that?"

Even worse, medication didn't seem to help. This clear pattern of procrastinating to one's own detriment did not yield to a simple upwards adjustment of the stimulant treatment. The search for the optimal balance between beneficial effect and adverse side effects, which is known as the therapeutic ratio, is what a good clinician would be expected to do as part of the treatment process. But beyond a certain dose of ADD medication, there is very little benefit and a near inevitable increase in unwanted side effects. With a larger dose, attention might improve but the capacity to "start, continue, and complete" was no better. And the patients were frustrated. Worse, they weren't coming back to my office and telling me what a magnificent and astute clinician I was.

And I didn't have a foggy clue as to what to do.

CHAPTER 5

What is the pause button effect?

If you are an adult with ADD, or a parent with an ADD child, or someone who has a relationship with a person with ADD (sibling, spouse, significant other, etc.), you know that there are many more challenges one faces than just inattention. It may be hard to put finger on what's so hard but if you stop and think about the overall deficiency of the person with ADD, it is almost precisely that: they often cannot just "stop and think." It is as if they have a defective "pause button" on their own personal internal remote control. When faced with a situation requiring a decision, they cannot find and access and hit their pause button; they can't stop, assess the situation, think things through, weigh consequences, and then decide on a course of action. Instead, they ignore or avoid or overreact or underreact.

When educating patients or other physicians about this aspect of ADD, I often refer to the Attention Deficit Disorder challenge as "bad decision-making". And I emphasize the point that impulsivity, which frequently results in bad decision-making, can be "overt" (obvious) or "covert" (hidden).

Overt impulsivity is demonstrated by the kid who gets into fights in the schoolyard. It is clear in the person who interrupts others all the time. It is obvious. Covert impulsivity is the teenager who, when asked if he is going to do his homework, replies, "Later" (read: No, and stop bugging me about it). Or the adult who is aware that she should be working on an important task but continues to put it off knowing full well that doing so will put her job in jeopardy.

Overt is obvious. Covert is not obvious. They are both bad decisions. Often really bad decisions. They are both examples of the frustrating, self-sabotaging and self-defeating day-in and day-out, moment-by-moment dysfunction that ADD people experience. But since so many doctors only consider ADD when faced with a fidgety hyperactive jumping bean, most don't take notice of a patient's inability to stop and think, to hit their pause button, to refrain from saying the wrong thing at the wrong time.

This "decision-making" capacity, which is almost always impaired in ADD people, and my inability to effectively address the debilitating executive function deficiencies it results in, presented a huge challenge to me as a clinician. Put simply, my patients were not getting fully better. In many, it was "half-a-loaf" improvement; in some, it was just a few crumbs. As a determined clinician, this outcome sucked for me. Intuitively, I knew that there was a great deal more that could be achieved in patients with ADD. It didn't make neurophysiological biological sense that only the "attention" aspect could be accessed and treated in the brain.

Now let's step back for a moment. What would most people do in this situation, whether as the patient, the parent, or the doctor? They would use common sense. They would encourage the person who is suffering to try harder. It doesn't work. Or to eat more healthy foods. It doesn't work. Or to make a schedule and stick to it. It doesn't work. Or to get counseling. It doesn't work. Or to see an ADD coach. It doesn't work.

From a medication perspective, many doctors interpret the lack of response and the accompanying frustration the patient feels as a reflection of depression or dysphoria or anxiety and prescribe an antidepressant (usually an SSRI, such as Prozac or Celexa or Cipralex). This route rarely works either. Although the patient may experience some short-term relief as the antidepressant alleviates some anxious feelings, the decision-making executive function capacity remains impaired.

What else do people try? They try being critical of the ADD person. It doesn't work. They punish the ADD person. It doesn't work. The ADD sufferer becomes self-deprecating and judges herself more harshly. It doesn't work.

And then, finally, lots of people with ADD try street drugs in an effort to self-medicate. Legions of ADD people smoke marijuana; many swear up and down that "this is the only thing that works for me." They claim "it slows my brain down enough for me to be able to concentrate." It doesn't work.

I'm not forgetting about diet and naturopathic treatment

here. People, with great hope and more than a bit of research, also try to alleviate symptoms of ADD with natural supplements and Omega-3 fish oils. It doesn't work.

Now understand that I am not opposed to trying any of these options. From time to time, we hear an anecdotal story that gives us hope. Acupuncture. Green tea extract. Pycnogenol Multivitamins. We listen. We read up on it. Maybe we even try it. It doesn't work.

What is the common thread in this process of trying to find an ADD solution? It is reminiscent of the old saying about throwing enough feces against the wall until you find what sticks. Now, I am not a purist. I am a hard-core clinician who treats patients all day, every day. To that end, I often have said that I don't care what works as long as something works. But there is a unifying thread underlying everything that is tried and doesn't work. The exercise, though well-intentioned, feels random and contrived. It is without a basis for understanding, without a framework for achieving a result that is consistent, measurable, and replicable.

Unfortunately, as medical professionals, even we had no understanding of a treatment model for Attention Deficit Disorder. There simply appeared to be no scientific basis to even begin to comprehend and conceptualize what this condition was exactly, and why it was, and what could be done about it, if anything.

In the late 80's and early 90's, around the time that I was searching for potential treatment models and new approaches to ADD, I became aware of a new medication that was gaining prominence in the treatment of both depression and bulimia in the

United States. This medication, Wellbutrin, was generating a number of treatment outcome report letters to the professional psychiatric journals that I subscribed to. It appeared to have a different mechanism of action than other antidepressant medications. In particular, it targeted different neurotransmitters than the usual serotonin "me-too" antidepressants. That neurotransmitter was norepinephrine. It appeared, in these early reports, to have not only a different side effect profile (less nausea, less fatigue, less sexual dysfunction, no weight gain) but it also appeared to provide a different qualitative therapeutic response, albeit for depression. People experienced "more bounce to their step" and a certain enhancement of their general capabilities.

I was interested, more interested than I would normally be reading about a new medication because this was a new category of medication. It was a norepinephrine reuptake inhibitor, which works to make the norepinephrine neurotransmitter more available at the synapse, the critical meeting point between two neurons where chemical messages are transmitted. I felt a surge of hope. This might be a very helpful molecule to become familiar with in the treatment of ADD. Could it be a significant complementary augmenting agent to assist my stuck-in-the-mud patients?

But there were two stumbling blocks. The first and most significant problem was that it was not available to be prescribed in Canada. Just as the FDA in the United States has to approve every prescription medication, so does the Health Canada institution. Luckily, this problem was not insurmountable. Although current regulations on accessing medications in the U.S that are not yet approved in Canada are more stringent, there was a more laissez-faire attitude at that time. For patients who could afford to travel across the border, it was possible to obtain Wellbutrin.

The second obstacle was the same one that had plagued the field of Attention Deficit Disorder all along—the refusal to consider using more than one medication at a time, even though many combinations were being used in the treatment of depression. I felt that I had both a medical and moral obligation to at least consider utilizing a combinatorial approach to the ADD conundrum.

In the specialty world of psychiatry, there are psychiatrists who are known in the field as "early adopters." These are leading edge clinicians who, having researched a new medication coming into the marketplace, are first to prescribe it to patients who may benefit. The success or failure of the first 5-10 trials of a new medication by an early adopter often determines both his willingness to incorporate it as a frequently relied upon therapy and to share the positive experience with colleagues. As a result, such physicians are aptly referred to as Key Opinion Leaders (KOLs) as they help guide and shape the utilization of new medications by other physicians in their geographic area and field of specialty.

When I started the use of Wellbutrin with my patients, I hadn't yet heard the terms early adopter and key opinion leader. I just wanted my patients to start improving. I'm pretty sure back then I would have been thrilled and relieved if they could do even a little better. I wasn't expecting much more than that. Also, because

Wellbutrin was a new medication and because I was using it in a younger population (teenagers initially), I needed to start at a low dose and build it up over the course of the first few weeks.

As a clinician, when you first use a new medication that you may introduce into your daily clinical practice, the most likely candidate to start with is not necessarily the most obvious. The first to try the medication are the toughest cases, the most treatment-resistant patients you have. It is the patients you haven't had any success with who become your in-office treatment trial group. That's right. You start with the group of patients that is most likely not to have a successful treatment response, which in turn will make you, more often than not, conclude that the medication does not work.

So it was for a group of hard-to-treat teenagers and young adult university students that I started to combine a stimulant treatment and Wellbutrin. To track their progress, I had the patients and their parents report back to me every few days. For my part, I hoped for something, anything good to happen. I may have even prayed a bit.

And within the first 2-3 weeks, a remarkable thing started to occur. The majority of these first few difficult, intransigent, not-much-hope-here, chronically procrastinating patients, and their parents, reported on the combination of their stimulant medication combined with Wellbutrin as follows:

- "I cleaned my room; I've never done that before."
- "I studied for my test and I got an A."
- "My kid was a pleasure all week."

- "This was the kid I always knew was in there."
- "I've never seen her work on her essay by herself."
- "We didn't have any fights or arguments."
- "I never knew I could do so well."

From an outside perspective, there were huge positive changes. All of these patients had become nicer and more composed. They were making better decisions. Their time management was better. They had better self-control. They were, like the famous rejoinder of the old Bachman Turner Overdrive song, Taking Care of Business. They didn't have that edgy jittery quality that was so much part of the usual ADD psychological state.

As treating physicians, it's easy to get discouraged if our first efforts with a medication don't work or worse, are a colossal failure, but Wellbutrin appeared garner remarkable successes. So much so that when my first dozen patients reported on their progress, I was frankly a little surprised, even a little shocked. "Really, it was that much of a change? You really felt, all of a sudden, like you wanted to do more, do better, get more done?"

The results seemed too good to be true. One successful case makes sense. You can always tell an anecdote about a patient who had an amazingly lucky and unexpected response to a treatment trial. But what I was seeing was far too consistent and dramatic to be just a lucky one-off. There had to be more to this story. I had to find some framework, some conceptual model, to help me understand what had just happened.

It was as though I was back on the golf course. I have always been a terrible golfer, really terrible. A business partner used to joke that I could afford the green fees but I couldn't afford to play because of all the golf balls I would lose each round. But every so often, I would hit a good shot. The problem was that I couldn't hit two good shots in a row because although I was trying hard to line up each shot, I didn't really know what I was doing. I lacked a proper understanding of the mechanics, physics, and sequencing of body movements needed to reliably replicate one good shot after another. Nor was I capable enough to know how to correct my game if a shot didn't go well. I just didn't have a conceptual model to work with— and I was facing the same problem with ADD.

Still, I wasn't about to let all the wonderful good fortune of my patients' unexpectedly robust treatment response go the way of my abysmal golf game. It was time to figure out what was going on. And why.

And so, as I continued to treat more and more patients with my combinational protocol, I started to evolve an understanding of the underpinnings of Attention Deficit Disorder. The minority of my ADD patients, perhaps a quarter, has a kind of mild inattention without much impulsivity. They generally respond well to a single stimulant medication, properly tailored to a maximal therapeutic ratio. These patients did much better once treated because, I surmise, the stimulant medication increases the availability of the neurotransmitter dopamine. Most stimulants enhance the dopamine neurotransmitter, resulting in a brain more capable of sustaining concentration and alertness.

But the majority of my patients, the remaining three-quarters, has all that other stuff I've been emphasizing—problems with motivation, procrastinating too much, being impulsive, having trouble regulating what they say, what they eat, what they spend, and the problems go on. So by adding another medication that helped the norepinephrine neurotransmitter levels, I was finally getting some purchase on all decision-making executive function issues.

I was really starting to get somewhere. The results in ADD patients, although not 100% consistent, were still completely remarkable. I knew there would be further refinements to the treatment process and to the conceptual model and although I wasn't sure which direction those would take, one thing was for certain: I was galvanized into action.

CHAPTER 6

Was I on the right track?

The more time went on, the clearer it became that this "two-sided coin" aspect of Attention Deficit Disorder was a crucially important step in the understanding of the condition and building of a new and dynamic conceptual model. Moreover, this model lent itself to a very clear treatment protocol that eventuated into dramatically improved treatment outcomes. I was helping more and more people with not just better results but often transformational results, both quantitatively and qualitatively.

But what did I really have? I was not a scientist running a huge laboratory with scurrying minions in white lab coats doing my bidding. I was not a lauded university professor with fawning residents and interns doing my intake histories. Nor did I have a battery of blood tests and magnetic resonance images (MRI's) to flash onto a PowerPoint presentation. All I had, it could be argued, was a huge capacity for work and a willingness to take on the tougher cases that other specialists had given up on.

What I had, at best, was a theory. It was this: The dopamine neurotransmitter system (in ADD at least) was primarily responsible for the regulation of attention and that the executive function and self-regulation issues were primarily mediated by the norepinephrine neurotransmitter. My theory was derived from the careful clinical assessment and treatment follow-up of the patients seen in my office as well as thinking through the potential biochemical basis of what I was observing in them.

I knew I was way more right than wrong. But the history of medicine and especially the history of psychiatry is riddled with quacks and egomaniacs and well-intended wrong-headed self-styled experts who lead people down the garden path to a dismal end. That said, most advances and breakthroughs in medicine don't occur in pristine high-tech laboratories. Most are the result of the careful, often collaborative, efforts of physicians trying to achieve better results by stepping away from the same-old same-old thinking of the past by bringing forth new ideas and perspectives to consider.

There was one obvious weakness in my treatment model, however. It was the fact that I was implicating two different neurotransmitters in the same problem. From a common sense standpoint, we all know that most complex problems cannot be reduced to a single issue or etiology. But in medicine and in psychiatry in particular, our bias is toward discovering the most logical and heuristic solution to a problem, the single smoking gun, if you will.

As a psychiatrist, medical school training is key because it requires you to learn the basic sciences. Apart from the obvious ones—anatomy, physiology, and the rest—one has to become familiar with biochemistry and chemistry. In considering two important neurotransmitters, dopamine and norepinephrine, they appear to be two completely different molecular compounds. Even their names sound different. How could one even postulate that two such different compounds could be involved in the same ADD problem?

To find the link, let's go back to medical school basics. Often in metabolic processes in the body, one entity can be transformed, or broken down, into another entity by a long series of enzymatically mediated biological reactions or steps. But what of dopamine and norepinephrine? Would there be many steps that transform one into the other? Was it even possible?

In fact, that transformation takes only one step. Only one. The dopamine molecule, in the presence of the enzyme dopamine ß-hydroxylase, adds a single hydroxyl group (or oxygen atom bonded to a hydrogen atom) to the dopamine structure and—voila—you have a shiny new norepinephrine molecule. This scientific revelation is key to understanding the ADD picture. When you factor it in, there are a couple of important medical conclusions that are potentially groundbreaking. For one, Attention Deficit Disorder just may be predominantly a "binary code" processing of dopamine and norepinephrine. Also, it is validation for taking a multipronged combinational medication approach, making this form of treatment both logical and necessary in ADD patients.

Most often, treatment advances are made by a combination of trying to make sense of a series of observations, some trial and error, and then a constant revising of one's understanding of why change is occurring. I would love to tell you that my treatment model was arrived at in one aha moment. Rather, it was more like a thousand "What just happened?" moments strung together and then reassembled into a working operational entity. But, once you have such a model, you then have the basis upon which to road test what you are doing. In no small way, you start to understand what will work and what won't and why. And you can start to predict outcomes and use your model to test whether it accurately anticipates what will happen.

One such event occurred in the early 2000's. A new medication for the treatment of ADD in children and teenagers was brought to the marketplace with great fanfare. The medication, Strattera (generic name atomoxetine), was received with tremendous enthusiasm by the psychiatric and pediatric community. In fact, at the time, it was the most successful launch of a new psychiatric treatment in history.

What accounted for this tremendous initial reception? Strattera was marketed as the first "non-stimulant" in the treatment of ADD. More amazingly, the doctor world seemed to accept quite easily that the term non-stimulant meant something, even though it seemed akin to calling a pet a non-dog. But the real reason for this vast acceptance was the profession's aforementioned unease and ambivalence to using stimulants. The new medication label "non-stimulant" automatically relaxed physicians, allowing them to be much more accepting of the treatment.

But exactly what was this new medication? As it turned out, Strattera was initially developed to be a new antidepressant. During the clinical trials that a new medication must go through before it is approved for use in the general population, it did not work well enough as an antidepressant. In other words, the clinical trial results did not reach statistical significance. However, Strattera was approved for use in Attention Deficit Disorder. Likely, a sharp observer noted a clinically significant improvement in a number of ADD symptoms and as a result, subsequent trials in ADD patients did achieve significance.

So what exactly is Strattera? More than a non-stimulant, it is a norepinephrine reuptake inhibitor. In common parlance, that means it enhances the availability of the norepinephrine receptor thereby enhancing executive functions. It helps with planning, time management, prioritization, reading social cues and motivation and helps to decrease procrastination. It also enhances the availability of dopamine but only a little.

Before Strattera came to be available for doctors to prescribe, I made the following prediction: Strattera would have a very eager and receptive response from patients and doctors alike because "non stimulant" treatment options would allow them to avoid the tarnished specter of using controversial stimulant medications. People all over would make a dramatic pronouncement that they were throwing the stimulants into the trash. Then they would warmly embrace, without the ambivalent feelings they had with stimulant medication, this new preferred ADD treatment.

I also predicted that within 6-9 months, children and teenagers taking the medication would be better behaved and generally nicer to be around but would be less focused and would experience a significant downward slide in their academic capacity secondary to a lesser ability to sustain focus and avoid easy distractibility. And that after a report card or two of failing marks, parents would declare the treatment a failure, discontinue Strattera, and return to stimulant medication. There would follow a period of improved school marks with the attendant improvement in focus and concentration but there would also be deterioration in behaviour and cooperation because there would no longer be sufficient norepinephrine support for the executive function/decision making/self-regulatory function side of the equation.

The final part of the prediction was depressing. With only half-baked results with separate treatment—either stimulant or non-stimulant—the parent or patient would declare that "nothing works" and ADD treatment would be abandoned altogether.

At that time, because of my prior experience with Wellbutrin, and because I had developed a conceptual understanding of Attention Deficit Disorder along with an accompanying treatment model, you can probably guess what I was doing in my office. For children and adolescent patients who needed improvement in their overall executive function, I combined the stimulant medication, which was enhancing the dopamine mediated improvement in the ability to focus and screen out distractions, with the Strattera, which was enhancing the norepinephrine mediated improvement in procrastination and motivation issues. And, lo and behold, I was getting great results—because finally, *both sides* of the ADD coin were being addressed.

Moreover, by starting at low doses and carefully adjusting the doses upwards, watching for the balance between effect and side effect, not only was the combination of stimulant (Concerta, Adderall or Biphentin) and Strattera effective, but it was very well tolerated. There were no significant drug-drug interactions.

Unfortunately, the academic centres, which most clinicians in private practice take their lead from when new treatment protocols are brought forward, categorically refused to consider this combinational approach. As in England of older times, the thinking was: "It is just not done." Despite how obviously helpful this new approach appeared to be, the strict confining orthodoxy of the academic world prevailed.

To make matters even more frustrating, at that time, the field of clinical psychiatry for adults was embracing the idea of combining medications into a treatment protocol to attempt to improve the results for mood disorders such as depression and bipolar disorder. Although I understood that the rest of the profession was many years behind my use of combining stimulants with Wellbutrin, a drug that was not an "on-label" identified treatment for ADD and was not approved formally for use in people under the age of 18, Strattera was not burdened by those two issues. It was "approved" for children and teens and it was "on-label". Considering this combinational approach shouldn't have been seen as outrageous, but it was.

So I had a very unusual and, for me, characteristic conundrum. I was helping a lot of people achieve heretofore unimagined improvements in their overall treatment results while at the same time being vilified by colleagues as a quack and by gossip mongers in the community as a pill-pushing madman. I was living in the world of topsy.

As all of this negativity was swirling around, I made an observation about the drug Strattera, which appeared to have too many patients suffering from significant side effects. I advised the drug company that makes Strattera that the dosing schedule appeared to be wrong. Many clinicians, particularly pediatricians who properly followed the drug company's dosing guide (start with 50% of the target dose and increase every 5-7 days to the target dose), ended up with almost half their initial patients suffering from severe stomach pain and vomiting within the first week. As a result, many clinicians swore off Strattera, which was gaining the reputation of a bad medication. I believe the drug company's concern was that if the dose wasn't increased quickly then patients and their parents wouldn't see results and Strattera may not be seen as effective as stimulant medication, which can work within days of the first dose.

This was misguided thinking for two reasons. Firstly, patients are told that this medication needs to be introduced to the body over 2-3 week period so as to "fly under the radar" of the body's side effect responses. Secondly, and more ironically, Strattera starts working quite well in most patients within a 10-14 day period even at low doses. Once the "direction" of the treatment is positively oriented, people are quite accepting of the start low/go slow approach of dosing. At that time, the drug company ignored my advice (perhaps because it was given for free).

Ten years later, though, after Strattera had hit the market, a clinical research study at an academic center in the United States proved my ADD thesis. The researchers had taken a group of child patients and treated them for 6 weeks with Concerta (once daily long-acting Ritalin) and observed their clinical response. Then they stopped the Concerta and started them on Strattera for 6 weeks and observed their clinical response. Then, after a couple of further weeks on no medication (a "wash-out period"), they placed the same patients on a combination of Concerta and Strattera. And guess what pleasant surprise they found? The children taking both medications at the same time did vastly better than they did on either of the medications on their own.

Who'd have figured?

CHAPTER 7

How does failure help us?

The practice of medicine is an exercise in repetitive humility. As a physician, one experiences failure as a regular part of every day. Even when you are good at what you do. Even when you are superb at what you do. Unfortunately, some failure is unavoidable and it always feels complete and bitter. The key to failure in medicine, though, is to learn something from it. More particularly, the treating physician needs to be able to both hate failure and at the same time, incorporate it into a more mature understanding of the real life limitations that medical practice imposes.

Failure can and should be a teacher. Seen in a positive, practical light, it can be a clue, a new language to be deciphered, a signpost pointing you in a different direction or toward a novel method of understanding. Failure is even more helpful if the clinician doesn't give in to feeling beaten down and resigned to it. We all know that in the end, we learn more from failure than success.

Which leads me to my feelings of failure. The problem with

my brilliant conceptual understanding of ADD and the dazzling treatment model I was constructing wasn't that it didn't work. The problem was that it didn't work all the time. And when it didn't work, when I failed to "deliver the goods" to the patient with ADD, it rankled. Badly. Not that I always expected to be successful in treating every patient. But when my treatment, based on my working model, failed, it wasn't just that I worried that the patient was not doing well. The failure also threw into question, and worse, doubt, whether I had any clue as to what I was doing. Like a big league professional baseball starting pitcher, I was only as good as my last outing.

So patients would come in for a diagnostic assessment and I would educate them on the treatment process and protocol. They would report back on their progress and would be seen in follow-up appointments. If they were doing very well, I would continue their treatment and maintain and monitor. If they came back and reported they were much more attentive but were still plagued by their procrastination/motivation issues, I would embark on the second part—Stage II—of treatment, utilizing a norepinephrine enhancing medication. They would then report back by phone within a 5-10 day period and would be seen two weeks later in follow-up. They would then report on their progress and the degree to which they felt their difficulties were improving or were even, possibly, resolved.

Now the degree of success that I have in treating patients with Attention Deficit Disorder was then, and continues to be, outstanding. So many people afflicted all their lives were, with treatment, reporting that they felt remarkably better. So much better, in fact, that I began to think it was just a matter of time until Oprah herself came by to offer congratulations and interview me about what I had discovered.

But still, a number of people would return after the Stage II trial and say that it didn't help—even if they lined up with the two-sided presentation of attentional difficulties and executive function deficiencies. I was thwarted in my steady march to Valhalla. I was baffled. Why wasn't my treatment working all the time?

Now, let's consider an analogy here. What we call Attention Deficit Disorder is really a cluster of described symptoms. In other words, by diagnosing someone with ADD, you are telling them: You have a sufficient number of symptoms that fit this entity's pattern. It is akin to going to the emergency department with crippling sudden onset stomach pain and being diagnosed with "abdominal pain disorder". The diagnosis is not specific enough and not very helpful. It doesn't even guide treatment. The fact is, the real problem could be gastritis or kidney stones or appendicitis or cancer, or a thousand other specific conditions with a dozen etiologies—inflammation, infection, tumor, obstruction, circulatory insufficiency, and the list goes on.

In psychiatry, we have to run with what we have, so to speak. So while I wasn't helping everyone, it was clear that I was still getting way better results and a vastly higher qualitative result than my colleagues were. And so, why was I so concerned about the few who weren't being helped? Accept your limitation. Accept the limitations of the state of the profession. Right?

Maybe I should have taken that approach. After all, I had done more for my patients than anyone else that I knew locally or internationally. And hadn't I been through enough already? Trust me on this: There is no financial incentive in medicine to become outstanding in your field. At the end of the day, quality doesn't get rewarded with money. Bad, useless, lazy, incompetent, and uncaring physicians can be much more financially successful than earnest, caring and committed ones.

What disturbed me most were the few patients who returned to the office and reported that not only did the Stage II treatment not work, but they felt worse off since the treatment began. Some couldn't sleep. Others were agitated "like I'm on crack." Others felt their mood worsen.

No one medication works for every patient. Every doctor knows that. But it was striking to see the same pattern over and over in the minority of patients for whom the Stage II treatment didn't work.

At that point, the most responsible and responsive thing to do as the treating physician would be to stop the second part of the medication treatment. Most of these patients had already improved their attentional issues with the use of stimulants. To use some clichés, half a loaf was better than none. You can't turn a sow's ear into a silk purse (now that's an old saying that dates me). Leave well enough alone. But still, it was frustrating because many of these patients should have fallen into step with the two-sided pattern.

What I would sometimes do, after waiting a few weeks to

allow the patient to settle, was initiate a trial with the alternative norepinephrine enhancing medication Strattera. And very occasionally, the expected Stage II result would emerge. Every person is unique and some medications will work in the same patient that similarly aimed treatment had not.

But most of the time, for this group of patients, success didn't come. And when it didn't, I was no further along in my understanding of why. And, if I figured the why part out, could I do anything about it?

In medical training, we are taught about the dose response curve, sometimes referred to as the "inverted U" or the "upside-down U". What this references is that most of the time, if a little dose is helpful and one continues to crank up the dose higher and higher, the previous good response starts to deteriorate and in fact worsen. In the accompanying graph, the idea is to try to hit the area of the dotted box—the so-called therapeutic window—with treatment. Too little of a dose is not helpful enough. Too much of a dose makes things worse.

This "inverted U" response is particularly striking when considering the effect of norepinephrine in the workings of the brain. If our central nervous system has too little operating norepinephrine, we become sluggish and lazy and inept. If we have too much circulating norepinephrine, we become agitated, fearful, and irritable. It is the middle zone we are trying to find.

Now let's return to my "failure"— the patients with the norepinephrine enhancing treatment who had become agitated.

Somehow, my adding in a medication that increased the availability of norepinephrine in the central nervous system was causing these patients to have "too much" norepinephrine.

Now remember that these patients were almost identical in their "two-side-of-the-coin" presentation as all the patients doing extremely well on this course of treatment. Quite clearly, the concept of "lifting" the level of dopamine with stimulant medication to help attention and then, for those patients who needed a second treatment to boost executive functioning, "lifting" their norepinephrine level, was not an effective model for everybody.

Around the time I was puzzling through this conundrum, a new medication hit the market. It was in the category of "atypical antipsychotics."

Figure 1

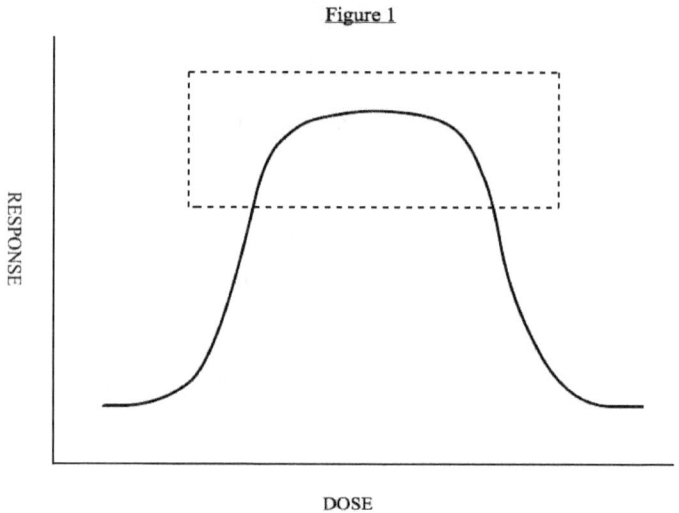

DOSE

These "more modern" medications, which assist people with serious psychiatric illnesses, such as schizophrenia, manic-depressive illness (also known as bipolar illness), and severe depression, are called atypical antipsychotics. As compared to the older "typical antipsychotic" medications, they have a less side-effect laden profile. In particular, they are much less likely to cause muscle stiffness and rigidity, an impassive mask-like facial expression, and long-term tardive dyskinesia (involuntary muscle movements). The classical picture of the chronic schizophrenic patient treated with long-term typical antipsychotics is the person sitting alone in the park who, from a distance, appears to be eating something. As you come closer, you see a constant mouth movement in a large chewing motion, which they have no control over. This is the so-called "rabbit mouth syndrome" (buccal-lingual syndrome is the medical term).

Atypical antipsychotics are not without risk. In particular, they are generally associated with a number of significant side effects, which require careful consideration. The most commonly known atypical is the medication Risperdal (also known as Risperidone). Separate for its use in high doses for severe psychotic illnesses, it gained a great deal of cache over the past 20 years as an adjunctive medication used in low doses for depression, anxiety, and behavioural disorders, particularly in children and teenagers. The major side effects are sedation and fatigue, increased appetite and weight gain, and an increased risk for metabolic syndrome.

Metabolic syndrome is a very concerning triad of increased weight (and risk for obesity), increased blood pressure (and consequent risk for developing hypertension or high blood pressure), and increased insulin resistance (leading to greater risk for developing diabetes). Not to be taken lightly, this risk develops over a period of months and even years.

In the early to mid 90's, Risperdal became a well-intentioned treatment for children and teenagers with severe behaviour disorders, including ADD and Oppositional Defiant Disorder (ODD). Because of its sedating "calming-down" effect, which could be seen within a few days, its use became widespread. Ironically, because of the "bad stimulant" mythology—how can you use stimulants in children? — many remarkably safe stimulants were shunned while Risperdal, which carried far greater long-term risks, was broadly used and even embraced. For some reason, these Risperdal medications were seen as a reasonably safe and effective choice for behaviourally troubling children with ADD over a multi-year span.

At the time, I raised the alarm about the longer-term use of Risperdal in children. Colleagues of mine were bemused, particularly in light of my well-known reputation for being on the leading and controversial edge of using combinations of medications in the treatment of Attention Deficit Disorder. But I said then, as I say now, that the modern understanding of ADD does not advocate the profligate and cavalier use of multiple medications in a ham-handed way. On the contrary. It is the very act of having a proper treatment model that allows for a deeper and broader understanding of how medications work and interact within the human body that should guide us.

My warning remained unheeded. More than 15 years ago, I said many times in speaking engagements: If you believe you can use an atypical antipsychotic with all the usual attendant side effects for many years in children and teenagers while discounting metabolic syndrome consequences as patients enter young adulthood, you are dreaming in Technicolor. And unfortunately, my prediction was right. Those side effects are precisely what emerged in the unfortunate pattern of long-time Risperdal use in young patients.

So clearly I was not an advocate of using the usual atypical antipsychotic. But there was a hugely important exception that emerged in my practice—and that was my utilizing a unique member of that group as an important component of ADD treatment. The exception is a medication called Abilify.

But wait, you say. Aren't you advocating using the very thing you were just condemning? Isn't Abilify a potentially harmful atypical antipsychotic?

In fact, though Abilify is lumped in with the atypical antipsychotic family, it should be in its own category because it has a completely different mechanism of action. All the atypical medications are "dopamine antagonists". That means that they sit on top of the dopamine receptor and block the connection between the dopamine neurotransmitter and the dopamine receptor.

Abilify, on the other hand, is a "partial agonist". This biochemical term means that sometimes Abilify acts as a dopamine blocker (antagonist) and sometimes as a dopamine receptor facilitator (agonist), stimulating and enhancing dopamine transmission. Not only is there a critical difference in its mechanism of operation but it also leads to a totally different side effect profile and dramatically changes the long-term risk profile. Unlike other atypical antipsychotics, which are usually taken just before bedtime in hopes that the sedative side effect helps patients sleep so they are not tired in the mornings, Abilify is generally taken in the morning to lift energy and mood. Also, Abilify is generally weight-neutral at low doses (in contrast to most atypicals) and so it does not cause unwanted weight gain.

Moreover, Abilify is the only true "neurotransmitter modulator". Effectively, it raises neurotransmitter levels in the brain if they are too low and lowers them if they are too high. The bottom line impact is to compress these levels into the Goldilocks middle where neurotransmitters work best, which takes us back to the "inverted U".

So I started to treat some cases differently. When a patient came back after the Stage II treatment was used to try to enhance the availability of norepinephrine and it hadn't worked or had gotten worse, I stopped the Stage II Wellbutrin and placed the patient on a low dose trial of Abilify instead. Within 1-3 weeks, these patients would return to my office and report three things to me.

First off, they reported feeling better, which wasn't surprising. Abilify at low doses is widely utilized to augment antidepressant response.

The second observation they reported was more interesting: I am *doing* better. The explanation? "That executive function stuff you were talking about, Doc, now it's really working. I am not procrastinating nearly as much, I'm more organized, my time management is so much better. Why didn't you have me taking this before?" When I first heard this positive response, I had to stop patients to ask, "Are you sure that's happening?" Because I hadn't expected it. Certainly Abilify was not a direct norepinephrine enhancer. But, as a neurotransmitter modulator, maybe it had taken the patient's adequate and sufficient supply of existing norepinephrine and had compressed, from above and below, the neurotransmitter level into the effective zone where it could now work properly.

The third news was also surprising. The patients would conclude their stories with "and I feel normal." I would joke with them and ask, "How do you know what normal feels like?" and they would answer, "I know it when I feel it."

Feeling better. Doing better. Feeling normal.

Now, with so much failure behind me, I felt I was really on to something. And I had discovered Abilify, another amazing medication that would help so many patients feel better than they ever had before. There was no doubt about it. My treatment model was starting to really hum.

CHAPTER 8

What do my patients say?

As I have explained, Attention Deficit Disorder remains poorly understood by the majority of adult psychiatrists to the point where, diagnostically speaking, it is "shunned" as a condition. As an active treating clinician, I am constantly surprised and disappointed when I see yet another adult patient with a painfully obvious ADD presentation whose life has been adversely impacted because of the condition's "non-diagnosis, non-treatment" status. To help convey a more clinical sense of the frustration ADD people experience, I have included a written history from a patient, a 46-year-old man working as an office manager in the financial services industry. His is just one example of the classic case of Adult ADD I see all the time.

"I am unable to focus. I find myself constantly distracted in my day-to-day life, particularly when I am working on mundane tasks. Example of this: I am unable to create and stick to a budget. I often forget commitments and conversations I have had with people. I have difficulty managing and estimating my time, which results in tardiness and the accompanying stress of being late or

missing appointments. I find it difficult to maintain focus throughout the life cycle of a large project. This means that the project is either not completed or is rushed through at the last minute and, consequently, is of mediocre quality. I find it difficult to relax on the weekend, often feeling that I have to be doing something.

Academically, I have seemingly always had behavioural problems: unable to sit still, blurting out answers, talking at inappropriate times. From elementary school and onward, I was frequently disciplined and spent a lot of time in the office. As I progressed into high school, I started skipping a large quantity of classes. I was able to get average grades (B average), but I knew I was capable of achieving higher marks. When I graduated from high school, I went to university. After my first year of university, I was kicked out due to poor grades. I went back after taking a year off and was again kicked out due to poor performance. I finally returned a third time and completed one year at Carleton University, where I did very well. I then returned to University of Toronto to complete the final two years of my degree. I was able to graduate with distinction. Following university, I went to chef's school where I completed the first of a two-year program. Following a stint as a chef, I returned to school at Industrial Training Institute where I completed a 6-month diploma in software development.

From a professional standpoint, I have been unable to stay in one career for more than five years. I have worked as a chef, software developer, business analyst, waiter, restaurant manager, restaurant owner, investment advisor, associate investment advisor, and assistant branch manager. I feel that I am capable of excelling in any of these careers, but I have tremendous difficulty setting long-term goals and working toward them.

When I was kicked out of university for the second time, I went to see a therapist. I was depressed and suffering from extremely low self esteem. I was never prescribed an antidepressant. I went for weekly talk therapy sessions. I stopped after about 18 months. I returned briefly to see the same therapist about two years ago when my career as an advisor started to suffer.

As far as what has worked for me… When I returned to university and had success, I found that doing things immediately when they were assigned was helpful. I had to avoid letting a number of assignments accrue; otherwise, I found the task of completing them all too daunting. I usually try to compile daily lists of tasks I need to complete to keep me focused. The problem I am experiencing is that I am not maintaining the system. As a result, tasks are not getting completed or are forgotten altogether. To give you a sense of how bad this has become, I have had to stop writing about a dozen time to look at my phone, check my email, etc."

As you can see, all of the hallmarks of what I have been describing are captured in this patient's description of his life to date. Like many adults, he was not overtly hyperactive as a child. What he had in spades, though, was the "two-sides-of-the-coin" feature—huge difficulty regulating his attention over the course of the longer day combined with disabling lapses in his executive function (procrastination/motivation issues). Yet he was well-dressed, impeccably groomed, well-spoken, articulate, and personable. Still, it is not surprising that he had so far not been diagnosed. I even told him that should he want to "road test" the matter, he could get assessed by nine more psychiatrists but I predict I would be the only one to tell him he needed treatment for Attention Deficit Disorder. The rest would zero in on his "mixed picture" of "depression and anxiety". And they would all be incorrect. Why?

In large part, they would be wrong for a very simple reason:

their education. They would all have been trained as adult psychiatrists. With little exception, for the past 40 years, whatever ADD training existed in the field of medicine in the area of psychiatry was offered in the subspecialty of child psychiatry only.

As noted earlier, psychiatrists are educated in the field of adult psychiatry with only a brief few months of training in child psychiatry. Within that very short hospital-based child psychiatry rotation, the psychiatry resident is burdened with having to learn the basics of an entire field of study. Attention Deficit Disorder would frequently not even show up on the radar screen during that time. Even residents choosing to subspecialize in Child and Adolescent Psychiatry were taught little about the nuts and bolts of properly assessing Attention Deficit Disorder. The neglect of such a crucial aspect of the field stemmed partly from a sheer pompous ignorance while another part was likely the result of the in-hospital emphasis of child psychiatry training versus the day-to-day clinic outpatient aspect of child psychiatric practice.

In any event, it has been only the truly exceptional adult psychiatrist who has emerged with anything more than a passing familiarity with ADD as a clinical entity. Rarer still, would be finding an adult psychiatrist with sufficient clinical expertise to approach using ADD medications with any comfort or facility.

To be fair, a truly good doctor, or any professional for that matter, is one who knows his or her limitations. If you aren't familiar with ADD medications and you don't know how to go about approaching the treatment, then far be it from me to criticize. But there exists a deep flaw in medicine and psychiatry. Doctors hate not knowing stuff. What they hate more is their patients figuring out that they don't know stuff they should know. So over and over, I see patients who have seen multiple professionals but never seem to get the proper diagnosis and treatment because the doctor willfully ignores the problem or worse, claims the patient has misinterpreted symptoms and is really just suffering from low self esteem or neurotic anxiety instead of ADD.

There is a central conundrum in the system itself, however, when it comes to Adult ADD. Adult-trained psychiatrists don't know much about Attention Deficit Disorder at all. Child-trained psychiatrists know, or should know, about ADD but mainly don't see adult ADD cases. And for many decades, ADD was taught only as a child's disease. Adult ADD was believed not to exist. So where does that leave all of these adult patients who are suffering every day?

As I became more involved in the diagnosis and treatment of ADD in a more complete and comprehensive manner, I came face-to-face with a long-standing dilemma. The vast majority of psychiatric medications are not "on-label" for children. That means that the various medications were tested on adults and subsequently approved for adults only. So historically, child psychiatrists who were willing to treat children and teens had to summon their courage and clinical skill to "borrow" from the adult compendium of medications in the treatment of their under-18 patients. This practice is known as using a medication "off-label".

The active clinical treatment of children and adolescents with

ADD required the clinician to utilize off-label treatments every day. In many ways, doing so is an extra burden that child psychiatrists shoulder if they want to achieve robust treatment results. It often is the distinguishing feature between a skilled experienced clinician and one who is content to only "do things by the book", to only use medications that are approved. It remains a sad fact that the major children's teaching hospital where I practice continues to use Prozac as their "first-line" (and often only line) treatment for depression and anxiety in their young patients because it is the only antidepressant "approved" and "on-label" for children and teens—simply because, as the oldest antidepressant in its group, it was the only one formally studied. The fact is, a quick survey of experienced clinicians in private practice would reveal that Prozac is rarely used as the first-line treatment for that age category because it has a higher likelihood of more adverse side effects than many other antidepressant medications and frequently causes agitation in children.

In other words, it is common for child psychiatrists to use adult medications in an off-label way for their patients, which leads me to the next refinement of my treatment model.

In the past few years, a new medication has gained "on-label" approval for children and teenagers in the treatment of Attention Deficit Disorder. This once-daily formulation of a short-acting medication called Guanfacine (trade name Tenex) had been around for many years in the United States although not available in Canada. The long-acting formulation, named Intuniv XR, allows the medication to be taken once daily (instead of three times) allowing for more convenience and a greater likelihood of maintaining its use. By the time it came out in Canada in 2014, it had already been available for three to four years in the U.S. Its availability was a milestone. It marked the first time that an ADD medication was approved for use as a potential add-on to the pre-existing stimulant treatment for ADD. It could be used on its own but its highest best use was in combination with a stimulant.

What is Intuniv XR exactly? First, let me tell you what it is not. It is not a psychostimulant, which would enhance attention, focus, and concentration. It is not in the antidepressant realm. It is not in the atypical antipsychotic group. Rather, it is in a category of older anti-high blood pressure medications called the alpha-2A agonists. What does that have to do with ADD symptoms? It has nothing to do with its anti-hypertension or blood pressure lowering impact. For people with ADD, it does something quite amazing: It has the ability to facilitate the transmission of dopamine and norepinephrine mediated signals through the frontal lobes of the brain.

The frontal lobe—everybody has two, one right, one left—is the seat of judgment, planning and decision-making in the brain. I sometimes refer to it as the executive function engine of the brain. It is where the "pause button" operates, the mechanism that allows people to stop and think and weigh consequences and options, all in milliseconds. Its effect is similar to a car's engine that gets its faulty transmission fixed thus leading to greater efficiency and output. In a nutshell, Intuniv XR allows for smoother, faster transmission of the neurotransmitter signals in the frontal lobes.

When that occurs, parents of ADD kids notice. After treatment, they return to my office 2-3 weeks later (it takes 10-14 days to start working) and report one or more of the following 5 frontal lobes mediated observations about their children:

1. Their thinking is sharper.
2. They are more productive.
3. They are more composed.
4. They are getting their act together.
5. They are nicer to be around and/or easier to get along with at school and at home.

There are additional benefits as well. Unlike the stimulants that work for a certain number of hours and then fade, Intuniv works around the clock. As a result, it helps the ADD patient in the morning before the stimulant kicks in after breakfast and in the evening as the stimulant effect wanes.

This drug has minimal side effects, essentially fatigue in some children and the chance for feeling light-headed on getting up quickly from a sitting or recumbent position, due to its momentary decrease in blood pressure called postural hypotension. Both side effects are generally easily managed. I usually initiate Intuniv XR in the evening so that, if it does cause some fatigue, it assists with sleep. The postural hypotension is generally transient and rarely leads to having to stop the medication.

It is also easily dosed. Most patients start with 1 mg for the first week or two and increase by 1 mg every 2 weeks as needed (always balancing benefit with side effect). The dose range is between 1-4 mg. Most of my child patients are on 2-3 mg tabs.

The weakness of Intuniv XR is the weakness of most medications. It doesn't work for everybody. In general, I have found this drug helpful in 6-7 out 10 patients. It can be utilized as a stand-alone treatment, as in the relatively infrequent cases of children and teenagers who either do not respond to stimulant medication or are exquisitely sensitive to side effects. However, as a stand-alone treatment, the results are clearly inferior than when it is more properly deployed as an augmentation strategy.

Where Intuniv XR has been very helpful is where it is also controversial—in the treatment of adults. In this case, which is the exception to the rule in ADD circles, the medication has not been formally studied in the adult world. But after a career of being forced out on a limb to "borrow" adult-approved medications for children, I was not about to allow others to browbeat me into not using a medication that could have an important role in the treatment of adult ADD symptoms, especially one that works so well, with minimal side effects and risk for drug interaction.

As I did previously with Strattera, I made an early prediction about Intuniv XR. Based on my understanding of it being a "facilitator" of neurotransmission, I predicted that it was very likely that the dose range used for child and teens (1-4 mg) was likely to end up being the same dose range for adults. My reasoning was straightforward. Like using a few drops of oil on your bicycle chain in the spring to help "facilitate" the gears, pouring more onto the chain has a rapidly diminishing rate of return. The chain's "transmission" has already been facilitated. I felt the same would be true with Intuniv XR—once facilitated, increasing the dose would yield little further benefit. And, with very rare exception, that result has been my experience.

One of my adult patients, who has enjoyed a robust response to the addition of Intuniv XR, was kind enough to share his experience. While not every patient will have the benefit of this result, this quote illustrates what is possible and emphasizes how the intelligent and selective use of psychopharmacologic intervention can assist ADD patients in achieving their full and true potential.

"The primary improvement I have noticed is that I somehow seem to be more intelligent. I cannot exactly explain how it happened, but shortly after I began regularly taking Intuniv (samples), I seem to have become more liked by my classmates and colleagues. I am now seen as an authority on many weekly class topics. People seem to want to work with me on class projects and are always inviting me to hang out with them after or outside of class. Of course, this may seem to be a common thing for fellow students to do, but it was always something that I had always been left out of (since I was young). Since I started my postgraduate degree (and Intuniv concurrently), things have changed for me. While I still have problems with attention, I am somehow now able to do all of my course reading and work at a much easier level than when I was doing my undergraduate degree. Essentially, my workload seems easier and I am doing better academically.

Interestingly, the above primary improvement had a secondary benefit: because I am doing better in my classes, I believe I am being perceived in a better light. Now my professors and fellow students often respect me because whenever a question or topic arises, I usually have answers or knowledge of them, perhaps because I managed to do all of the readings. This is something I find hard to explain, as I do not fully understand how I have come to be so well-regarded in such a short time. In my opinion, Intuniv has made my life better; my academic and personal life has taken off, as evidenced by how my accomplishments seem to be multiplying—often too fast and without trying.

Although I still experience problems, I can now reflect and consider my options before acting, which has always been something of a problem for me. I will continue taking Intuniv as long as I can access it because it has made such a positive impact on my life.

It should be noted that I feel no negative side effects from Intuniv. It also works well with my Adderall and Wellbutrin."

By now, you should have an understanding for this new way of treating Attention Deficit Disorder. To recap: Two sides of the ADD coin are mediated largely by two different neurotransmitters. You can increase the availability of dopamine to assist focus. You can then increase the availability of norepinephrine to assist executive function. You can then try to bring those neurotransmitter levels into the most optimal zone so the brain can operate with greater efficiency. And finally, if needed, you can augment the result by enhancing the smoothness with which the signals are transmitted through the important areas of the brain.

In these next few chapters, I am going to take you out of the "classroom" and into my office so you can get a "desk-side" view of what I do and how I do it, what I say to patients, and what protocols I have developed to achieve results on a day-in day-out basis. My hope is that this insider snapshot will offer a more practical perspective on the treatment model while providing a roadmap that you can follow along yourself.

CHAPTER 9

How do I know you have ADD?

Now, a confession. I am technologically challenged. I have never had any skill or facility with computers and modern technology. If there is a way to press the wrong button or mouse click on the thing that will wipe out all of your work, I seem to have an uncanny ability to find it. So I have made my peace with technology by generally avoiding it. The fact that I now belatedly have an iPhone and can, with assistance, negotiate through its various utilities with some facility astonishes my children.

Recently, I was completing a first assessment appointment with a professional technology executive in his mid-thirties who is vice president of a software company. As I made handwritten notes, he asked if I minded if he asked me a personal question. I told him I didn't mind. He then asked, "It's been a long time since I've been in an office that didn't have a computer. Why don't you have one?"

I replied, "Well, I've been doing this for a long time. And I'm pretty efficient with my old system. If I was starting my practice today, I'm sure I would be wired to the hilt but I'm not that interested in changing my approach now. My system can't really crash. And I have a concern that if I used a computer, I'd end up being less efficient, not more."

Without missing a beat, he said, "Oh for sure you would be less efficient."

I was taken aback as I was expecting the usual lecture about the wonders of modern software. So I asked him, "You are in the business of computers. Why would you say that?"

"Because a computer on your desk essentially represents a massive distraction all day long," he replied. "You wouldn't be able to be as focused on what you do."

You might be thinking that this is my opening gambit leading to a shrill warning about the dangers of our wired-up, "always on", smartphone-addicted society breeding an entire generation of attentionally challenged individuals with a concomitant spike in incidence of Attention Deficit Disorder. It is not. ADD existed for eons prior to the birth of computer and cell phone. My point is much simpler.

In order to assess an ADD patient (child or adult), one does not need scurrying minions administering multiple computer-guided tests. They do exist, and as new and refined procedures evolve, there may be a more defined role for them, but in the current state of the art, there is no single technology-based diagnostic assessment tool for Attention Deficit Disorder. I say that not because I am technologically behind the times, but rather, to offer encouragement to medical and mental health professionals who feel intimidated in developing greater expertise in the assessment and treatment of ADD.

Currently, many family doctors, pediatricians, and psychiatrists wrongly insist to their patients that in order to be diagnosed with Attention Deficit Disorder, they have to obtain a full psychological educational assessment. This assessment is comprised of two full days of testing by a registered clinical psychologist at a cost of two to three thousand dollars. The problem here, apart from the prohibitive cost to many patients and their families, is the fact that there is no single psychological test that is diagnostic of ADD. Nor is there a combination of multiple psychological tests that nails the diagnosis. (Note that this ADD assessment process is very different from the essential role that psychologists play in the delineation of other challenges, such as learning disabilities, for instance).

So how exactly should Attention Deficit Disorder be best diagnosed? A good clinician who can elicit a proper history while listening conscientiously to the historical narrative the patient provides is the single most important factor in the diagnostic process. Full stop. It's the key to proper diagnosis, regardless of computerized testing, so it's so important to learn about what to listen and watch for. As the doctor, people depend on you not to miss signs or worse, ignore them. So if you are the patient and your doctor doesn't know what they are observing when it comes to ADD, don't give up; take it upon yourself to get to a doctor who does.

When I am contacted for an assessment, I tell the patient to type three or four paragraphs outlining the problems and symptoms they are experiencing, what they've tried to do about them, what treatment they have had (if any), what has worked, what hasn't, and what they are hoping to achieve. These "mini histories" are remarkably helpful and are frequently very illuminating and often touching as well. Perhaps most importantly, they provide diagnosis-assisting information that helps shape the history taking of the consultation. I have selected a few of these personal summaries to share here.

Personal Patient Summary #1

"I am a 29-year-old and a year 5 PhD candidate at university. I have always struggled with focusing and paying attention to my work and have noticed a difference between procrastination and an inability to do my work despite my best efforts. During late winter/early spring 2014, I finally decided to see if there was something more to my struggles than just "lack of discipline" and found Dr. T who was able to help me determine that as suspected, ADHD might be a problem. I initially tried to bring the problem to my family doctor (I have since switched doctors) who dismissed my concerns as someone who "perhaps just needs to work a bit harder or change professions" since "everybody has trouble focusing and being a doctoral candidate was hard work".

In March 2014, Dr. T, based on available clinical data at the time, assessed that my DSM-5 diagnostic impression was: Adult Attention Deficit Hyperactivity Disorder, Predominantly inattentive presentation; Generalized Anxiety Disorder; Prominent Avoidant Traits; Dependent & Depressive Traits.

Which makes sense and explains quite a bit of my childhood, adolescent, and young adult life. I have since tried to introduce medication and therapy to my daily life in order to understand myself and become a more efficient and productive individual (when it comes to my career choices). In regards to therapy, I am admittedly inconsistent. Between balancing my finances and simply keeping track of time, I tend to introduce several month long breaks in between sessions. I am working on it. I am back in therapy with Dr. T. Medication has been more problematic.

When I switched to the new Family Health Team, I was introduced to Dr. S, who wanted to start me slow and targeted my anxiety first, and then wanted to put me on a non-stimulant for my ADHD. However, Dr. S left the practice early on in my treatment and I was switched to Dr. P, who I believed was not as dedicated to my treatment as Dr. S was. There were a few mishaps with my file and between my confusion and miscommunication between myself, my pharmacy and the doctor's office, I ended up being dosed with 100 mg of (generic brand) Zoloft and 100 mg (generic brand) Strattera. I was waking up with sweats, had night terrors and couldn't sleep at night and if I took the medication in the morning, it would make me fatigued by lunchtime. By then, Dr. P had moved to an office that I could not easily get to and I am now with Dr. M. I am no longer on my medication because I am pretty sure that was not what I was supposed to be taking. It was causing me problems and I was having trouble scheduling an appointment with a doctor who could see me at the Family Health Team.

The short of it is that I don't really understand how the medication is supposed to work. I am nervous about it, and know that in general, I am supremely sensitive to stimulants (such as caffeine) and am wondering if it will

translate to my response to the medication that treats ADHD. Dr. T suggested
that you would be able to help me with my treatment and also better help me
understand the medication side of things. So here I am. Thank you for your time.
I really appreciate it."

Personal Patient Summary #2

"Growing up, I was terrible at math and received average grades in
everything else. In high school, I had something called visual therapy to help and
I'm not sure of the outcome. In the 70's and 80's, ADD was not as widely
known and I did not receive any help. I just thought I was not that smart.
Average. After high school, I went to a women's college and studied Art History
and did really well because I was interested in the subject and had a lot of
attention. I then went on to interior design school and found my talent. After
graduation from college was when I decided to get tested for ADD. My two sisters
and one brother, who are much older, were having their children tested and treated
for ADD. I took Ritalin and Dexedrine. They were both effective but I did not
continue taking medication after a couple years. I just wanted to be natural and
accept my brain as it was. That was 20 years ago. Time files.

Now I'm 45 and at a point in my life where I feel like I need to step up
my game and really utilize my talents. I'm not living up to my potential. I am
very talented but cannot seem to get myself together to succeed. At times, I get in a
design frenzy where I am super-focused on making my surroundings look and feel
better and I ignore all other priorities.

I am constantly overwhelmed by mess and three children talking to me at
the same time. The after school activities, planning and homework are
overwhelming, leaving me grumpy and full of anxiety. I spend too much on

impulsive shopping; I cannot seem to conquer the task of regulating our finances.
Since I work from home, my family life and design life are all mixed together.

I can see a vision for what I would like my life to be like but I just can't
seem to reach it because of feeling overwhelmed by all the details. It's like I have it
all in my brain at the same time, all the time."

Personal Patient Summary #3
"Nature of the Problem

The nature of the problem is that I find it very hard to stay focused and
motivated while studying. Additionally, when I get to the library, I am focused for
a temporary period of time and then I find that my mind is wondering and I have
no motivation or focus to continue my studies. I find it frustrating that I can't
keep my mind from wondering, even when I'm determined to study. Nothing seems
to work. This has resulted in me rarely achieving productive work and it is only
adding to my frustration.

Symptoms

Some of the symptoms that contribute to this problem are my lack of
focus, no motivation, lack of desire to study, trouble managing tasks and my time
properly, I find I get bored easily and I get very easily distracted. Additionally, I
find it hard to sit still in one spot for an extended period of time (i.e. I feel the
need to get up and walk around).

How has it impacted me?

This has impacted my grades somewhat; I feel I could have achieved
better marks in university if I was more focused and motivated. I find that tasks
take me a lot longer to do because of how easily distracted I am and therefore, it
takes me a lot longer to complete my studies and assignments than originally

planned. I've been out of school, graduated, for two years and it has taken me over
a year and a half to finally start my accounting courses because of my lack of
motivation and desire to start the courses, even though I know it is something I for
sure want to do in my life. I find I am constantly procrastinating in life.

What do I want to get out of this?

I want to find something that will keep me motivated and focused in
order to accomplish my goals of becoming a chartered accountant and having more
focus, motivation, and determination in my day-to-day life. Additionally, I would
like the ability to not become distracted so easily so I can manage and organize my
tasks both in school and life."

Collateral history is very important in the overall assessment
of Attention Deficit Disorder. Getting the facts is obviously more
directly obtainable for children and adolescents because the history-
taking initial assessment is always done by an adult family member.
Still, other sources of history and observation do exist for adult
patients—siblings, friends, spouse and colleagues are often available
for information. In real-life practice, however, many adults who seek
a diagnostic consultation are reluctant to involve anyone else in the
process because of privacy and confidentiality concerns.

One excellent potential source of information, even in adult
patients, is to ask the patient to bring in a file of their old report
cards. Even if the patient doesn't have such a file, many of their
parents will still have a yellowing collection somewhere. Though it
sometimes feels like I am on an archeological dig, much information
can be mined from these troves. In particular, I am tuned in to the

"ADD-likely" clues that are regularly and reliably found in a patient's report card files. In particular, the phraseology of underachievement is rife—not working to potential, could do much better, needs to come to school with the right attitude. Issues of inattention abound as well—can't concentrate for longer, rushes through work just to get it finished, easily distracted. A wide scatter of marks is frequently seen, A's or D's, often reflecting whether the ADD patient was interested in the particular course or not. There is often a pattern of early success and high grades in the first few years of elementary school followed by a significant plummet in grades 6-8 when homework and assignment completion play a larger role. "Would have done so much better if assignments were handed in" is a report card red flag.

If psychological testing has been done, I ask the patient to make a copy for me to read and put into their chart. However, as noted previously, this piece is neither essential nor diagnostic.

Each of my adult patients also fills out the Adult ADHD Self-Report Scale (ASRS) Symptom Checklist (see below), which takes only a couple of minutes for most patients to complete and provides the clinician with an easy-to-use screening tool. While ADD kids can focus on favourite subjects quite well, I use this test to bring to light what happens when they are trying to work on subjects that don't interest them. In children and adolescent patients, I go through each of the 18 DSM-5 symptom questions below and request "yes/no" answers with "maybe" counting for half a point. I preface each question pertaining to being at school dealing with "not-your-favourite" class.

Adult ADHD Self-Report Scale (ASRS-v1.1) Symptom Checklist

Patient Name		Today's Date					
Please answer the questions below, rating yourself on each of the criteria shown using the scale on the right side of the page. As you answer each question, place an X in the box that best describes how you have felt and conducted yourself over the past 6 months. Please give this completed checklist to your healthcare professional to discuss during today's appointment.			Never	Rarely	Sometimes	Often	Very Often
1. How often do you have trouble wrapping up the final details of a project, once the challenging parts have been done?							
2. How often do you have difficulty getting things in order when you have to do a task that requires organization?							
3. How often do you have problems remembering appointments or obligations?							
4. When you have a task that requires a lot of thought, how often do you avoid or delay getting started?							
5. How often do you fidget or squirm with your hands or feet when you have to sit down for a long time?							
6. How often do you feel overly active and compelled to do things, like you were driven by a motor?							
							Part A
7. How often do you make careless mistakes when you have to work on a boring or difficult project?							
8. How often do you have difficulty keeping your attention when you are doing boring or repetitive work?							
9. How often do you have difficulty concentrating on what people say to you, even when they are speaking to you directly?							
10. How often do you misplace or have difficulty finding things at home or at work?							
11. How often are you distracted by activity or noise around you?							
12. How often do you leave your seat in meetings or other situations in which you are expected to remain seated?							
13. How often do you feel restless or fidgety?							
14. How often do you have difficulty unwinding and relaxing when you have time to yourself?							
15. How often do you find yourself talking too much when you are in social situations?							
16. When you're in a conversation, how often do you find yourself finishing the sentences of the people you are talking to, before they can finish them themselves?							
17. How often do you have difficulty waiting your turn in situations when turn taking is required?							
18. How often do you interrupt others when they are busy?							
							Part B

The Adult ADHD Self-Report Scale (ASRS-v1.1) Symptom Checklist was developed in conjunction with the World Health Organization (WHO), and the Workgroup on Adult ADHD that included the following team of Psychiatrist and researchers: Lenard Adler, MD, Ronald C. Kessler, PhD, Thomas Spencer, MD.

In the questionnaire, the 9 questions about inattention are the most crucial diagnostically. There are many adults who will have none of the 9 "hyperactivity impulsivity" symptoms and end up with a total score of 6-7 out of 18. But if those 6-7 are clustered in the inattention section, then the patient is still in the ballpark for ADD in my clinical experience.

When I take the history, I am particularly interested in establishing that there has been a clear and longstanding difficulty with sustaining concentration for longer periods, even if this problem was not apparent in earlier grades of school. Many highly intelligent people with ADD are able to compensate adequately for long periods, even through high school, but then "hit the wall" toward the end of that period or even later in post-secondary education.

Once concentration is observed, the next question I ask is about procrastination/motivation issues. In most people with ADD, the most frequent response comes with a chortle of self-recognition. "Oh my God, Doc, that is my biggest problem. I am the King (or Queen) of procrastination. If I could just get started and see things through to completion, I wouldn't be sitting here today. All my life, I always leave things to the last minute and then I get into a complete panic the night before."

These two aspects of a patient's history—concentration and procrastination/motivation —are the bedrock of the diagnosis. Certainly there are those occasional cases that present with just inattention (20% or so). But the majority of the cases that I see have both the dopamine-mediated inattention and the norepinephrine-mediated procrastination/motivation issues as the hallmarks of the symptom complex.

There is almost always a third aspect of the presentation as well, and that is a clear level of underachievement in comparison to their level of intellect. Almost all of my ADD patients have a kind of "coulda-shoulda-woulda" in their presentation. In other words, they are smarter than how they have performed. And they suffer with the frustration that accompanies these feelings: "Why haven't I done better? Why was I not in the lineup when the royal jelly was being passed out? Why haven't I done as well as friends that I went to school with?"

When I see that triad of inattention, procrastination/motivation issues, and underachievement to the level of intellect, my clinical sense is that the diagnosis is Attention Deficit Disorder until proven otherwise. Most of my colleagues would bend themselves into pretzels admonishing me for being too hasty and over-inclusive in the diagnostic process. And there probably should be a couple of modifying qualifiers added to my statement. But relatively speaking, particularly with the overwhelming reluctance of the profession to make the diagnosis and engage in a treatment process, the statement stands. It is Attention Deficit Disorder until proven otherwise.

What are some of the other important clinical clues that are strongly indicative of an ADD diagnosis?

The most important diagnostic "procedure" is the carefully

taken history. Of course, that is probably true of many medical and psychiatric assessments but even more important in the absence of all the other tests that doctors in other parts of the medical world rely on: physical examination of the patient, laboratory testing of blood, urine, and secretions, ultrasounds, MRI's, CT and x-ray scans. In the ADD area, it is the history that is the most important marker, including the crucial gathering of collateral history.

There are other important "red flags" that can aid in helping to consolidate the likelihood of an accurate diagnosis. I have already mentioned the frequent and striking feeling of the patient having underachieved to their intellect, the so-called "what is wrong with this picture?" presentation. What are some of the other ADD clues, particularly the major ones, that I look for in the history?

A telltale clue, as illustrated in Chapter 1, is what I refer to as "first-year university student collapse syndrome". I see this feature so often that I have come to the point that when I don't see it, I drill down harder with my history taking. The struggle that a young college age student feels inside an unstructured environment—living away from home, needing to be self-disciplined, needing to rely on oneself to initiate a task/project/assignment and see it through to completion by a deadline with no one "riding hard" on you—is a set-up for failure in many ADD cases. In fact, if staff members at colleges and universities were more aware of the enormity of this single factor in their student population—that of the undiagnosed and untreated first year student falling apart—they could dramatically improve their undergraduate retention rate by providing a more enlightened Student and Health Service component to support and treat this very large cohort.

A number of years ago, I was asked to speak at weekly rounds to the 17 psychiatrists that comprised the University of Toronto Psychiatric Health Service about "Attention Deficit Disorder in the University Age Population". As people filed in for their mandatory attendance seminar with less than polite enthusiasm, I sensed that this was not going to be the most open and receptive group. So, since I am clearly a graduate of the Dale Carnegie How-to-Win Friends-and-Influence-People course, I opened with the following statement: *"You are the University of Toronto Psychiatry Services. Young people come here from all across the country and from places farther away and they depend on you to help them, to shepherd them through tough times when they occur. And you are missing Attention Deficit Disorder all day long. And you are letting these young people down when you could be crucially important in setting them on the right track in life."*

I am happy to report that about half of the psychiatrists present started to think about ADD right away. And in the next few weeks and months, they started to treat it. The other half, as might be expected, still thinks I'm a jerk.

The point remains. If a person who appears intelligent tells you that he or she struggled badly in the first couple of years of university, you should be fully attuned to the likelihood of Attention Deficit Disorder. Don't fall into the easy trap of assuming "not grown up enough, drank too much, partied too hard, needed to sow their wild oats". That is all sloppy and clichéd thinking and it's not helpful to someone who is suffering and seeking help.

Another leading indicator of ADD can be found while taking the patient's history of drug and alcohol use. Many people will have tried to "self-medicate" their condition with marijuana and/or alcohol. They frequently describe that dope is the only and best thing they can do for themselves because, for a period of time at least, it slows down the rapid cascade of thoughts leading them to feel they are gaining greater clarity and control. In fact, they are not. Getting high and stoned does provide some sense of brief slowing but without sustainable clarity. It also causes thinking to soon become scrambled, interfering with effective studying, which requires memory to be laid down like train tracks in the brain. Plus, it steals motivation, which people with ADD already tend to lack.

One real clinical pearl that helps to differentiate the ADD individual is found by asking about cocaine use. If the answer is yes, I follow up by asking what effect it had. The overwhelming majority of patients respond something like this: "My friends got high and I went and cleaned my room. I was able to think and focus clearly in a way I never could before". As it turns out, this is a story that I hear so often that the more expected answer — "I got so high"— would give me pause with respect to an ADD diagnosis. That's because cocaine, albeit in non-therapeutic dosages, mimics the impact psychostimulants can have in the ADD brain, thereby creating the paradoxical effect of greater clarity and concentration.

When I ask about past treatment efforts by other therapists, psychologists and/or psychiatrists, and there is a recurrent history of non-response or only a partial transient improvement to properly administered cognitive behaviour therapy and serotonin-related antidepressant medications, that is another ADD red flag. There is no doubt that we in the mental health field try hard to get our patients better. And most of us are good at what we do. So when one sees, over and over again, people who have endured 4-6 failed efforts at therapy—psychotherapy and pharmacotherapy—but always end up in the "depression/anxiety" area, that is often because the doctor has failed to extend the diagnostic awareness to a different perspective. Without simplifying things too much, shouldn't we always ask whether this is depression or anxiety *or* self-regulatory dysfunction?

In the diagnostic process, one should always inquire about psychiatric difficulties in any family members. Attention Deficit Disorder, as it turns out, is much more inheritable than almost all psychiatric disorders. In fact, it is very common for an adult to seek out a diagnostic assessment after his or her child has been diagnosed. Even in the absence of a formal diagnosis of ADD in a parent or sibling (because ADD was almost never diagnosed in previous generations), a history of similar struggles with similar symptoms resulting in unhappiness, underachievement, frustration, and substance abuse is very common. "I'm sure my father and sister have this, too," is common currency in my office.

There are two more important distinguishing features of ADD. The "Mental Status" part of the assessment is a standard part of any psychiatric interview. "How is your mood?" or "How have you been feeling in the past few days and weeks?" is a common question that a psychiatrist will pose to the patient. ADD people will very frequently response with this type of answer: "Up and down" or "Really all over the place" or "My mood can change so quickly". To the inexperienced clinician, or simply one who has never stepped outside of the rigid box that psychiatrists frequently consign themselves to, these answers shout "bipolar disorder" (manic-depression) and/or "mood instability".

In fact, they are not indicative of these diagnoses at all. Real bipolarity requires a sustained clear mood change (either depressed or manic) that lasts several days, if not several weeks. With just a little more inquiry, the physician will discover that what the patient means is that they can have a short sharp change in their mood half a dozen times every hour. "I was feeling fine, Doc, and then that jerk in the desk next to me kept tapping their goddamn pencil! And I got really bugged. But then I settled down." Described in that way, the scenario is decidedly not a mood swing. What it does represent, though, is a relative inability to maintain a sense of being able to smoothly and regularly have one's own hands on the steering wheel of one's own life, of being able to confidently self-regulate.

Finally, people with Attention Deficit Disorder, in adulthood particularly, are often significantly overweight. It is not that they are constantly food seeking in a ravenous manner. Many will say, "I don't even pay attention to what I am eating; I don't even know what I put in my mouth." To someone who is simply weight conscious or even preoccupied with food, this statement sounds preposterous. It's not. ADD people not only do not pay attention to what they are ingesting, they double down on their weight-control problem by not paying attention to their satiety (enter that portion of our brain that send out signals telling us we are getting full or "sated") and that we should slow down and stop. Guess what happens over time when that pause button gets ignored? You got that right.

To recap, Attention Deficit Disorder is not a "lazy" problem. It is not a "you could do it if you wanted to" challenge. It is a disorder of self-regulation. And if you can't self-regulate, then good luck getting through life.

CHAPTER 10

What do I tell my ADD patients?

At the conclusion of the assessment consultation, I usually leave a few minutes to answer questions and discuss the process going forward. Most patients I end up seeing have already been through a long frustrating process of misdiagnosis and non-treatment. As a result, I always make clear that I have no intention of "letting grass grow under our feet." In this chapter, imagine you are sitting in my office in the patient's chair across the desk from me. As I am often talking with my hands, I will include the stage directions as needed so you get the full picture. While some of what I explain may seem redundant, remember that I aim to consolidate the entire educational component of the treatment model and approach. I do so because a better-informed patient is vastly more likely to be engaged in his or her own treatment as a full partner. Consequently, I have much better compliance with treatment trials in my patients because they haven't just been handed a prescription with the exhortation "try this" or "trust me." They know what's going on and why.

What I present here is no different than what I say when I give talks to doctors directly. I want you to know that I am not trying to "be nice to you" but rather I am intent on being accurate. Even though I am the doctor and you are in the position of patient, and we are discussing medication treatment, which is the "medical model of illness", keep in mind that Attention Deficit Disorder is not an illness. It does, however, have everything to do with function, similar to finding the reasons that a person needs glasses. You don't wear glasses because you have an illness of your eyes, an infection, inflammation, tumour, or cataract. You wear glasses to give your perfectly healthy eyes the opportunity to operate at the peak of their natural biologically intended functionality. Same goes for ADD.

As a result, I am going to try to fashion the best pair of "inside-the-head" glasses I can for you to allow your perfectly healthy smart brain the opportunity to operate at the peak of its biological functional capacity. Function, not illness. Full stop. No qualifiers.

As discussed, the problem that you have as an ADD patient can be looked at as a two-sided coin. One side of the coin is the regulation of attention. This lack of proper regulation does not mean that you can't pay attention. It means that you have a great deal of difficulty concentrating on something for an extended and sustained period of time, particularly if you are not interested or entertained by it. To be a good student, a person needs to be able to concentrate on subjects they like and on the stuff that bores them to tears. Then there is the decision-making side of the coin, or the executive function side. What that really references are the procrastination and motivation issues.

If you don't remember anything else about today's session, please take away the following. If you are smart to begin with (even though you, like most

ADD people, have probably reached the point where you are no longer too sure about your intellect), but you've got problems on this side of the coin (my left hand is flapping now) and on the other side of the coin (my right hand is flapping now) then, guess what, you've got problems. If you get this side of the coin (left hand flapping) fixed but you still have problems on this side (right hand) then you will do better but not that much better. If you get this side of the coin (right) fixed but you still have problems on this side of the coin (left), you will do better but not that much better. But if you get both sides of the coin engaged (both hands now flapping), the game changes. And you need game-changing treatment. Because without both sides of the coin treated, you will remain very frustrated and thwarted and always feeling that you are never going to be good enough.

If and when we start treatment, we are going to start on this side of the coin (left hand flapping). I am going to start you on a medication that is intended to significantly improve your focus and attention and maintain both through the course of the day. I will be giving you a prescription and an agenda which will take you through the first 7-8 days to a standard dose for size and age. You will call me a couple of times in the first 8 days to report to me that we are on the right track. Then we will meet again.

We take those first days to see if the treatment works. Then, if we are moving in the right direction, we will spend the next two weeks "tailoring" the dose—a little higher here, a little lower there. Then we will run with the tailored dose for two more weeks, and meet within that time to review your progress.

At the end of that 4-5 week period, we meet for a review session at which time I will ask how you are doing. A quarter of the people I see will come back and say, "Wow, I am doing so much better. More focused. I can concentrate for longer. I am more organized. I am getting more done. It's really great." You *have come by chance to be in this group.*

The other three-quarters of my patients, and most likely you, will come to the review session and tell me some variation on this theme. "Dr. Hoffer, I am more focused. I guess that is good but I am disappointed and underwhelmed. I really thought this was going to make a bigger difference in my life. But I still don't get things done. I don't start things I need to get going on. I still procrastinate like crazy. I'm not motivated like I should be. And how crazy is this? I used to think that I wouldn't procrastinate so much if only I could pay attention. But now I can pay attention reasonably well and I'm still procrastinating. That's why I'm so disappointed and discouraged."

For people who fall into that majority situation, I then start a session medication which works on the other side of the coin. I'll go into detail on that process in our next session. Suffice to say for now, that "Stage II" treatment only takes a couple of weeks to test. And if it works well, or even just indicates we are moving in the right direction, then the game changes or, at the very least starts to change.

We are not going to start today. It is so important for you to do this right that I don't want you to feel rushed. I am going to have you come back for an education session. In that session, I will go over what this is, what it isn't, how one conceptualizes the process, what are the medications, what are the side effects, what is the time frame and the agenda. By the time we are through, you will know more about ADD and how to understand it and how to approach the treatment of it than most doctors.

Consider this an education session, not a sign-up session. Some people, after completing the education session, will want to start treatment the next day. Others, who need time to digest it all, will say, "That's a lot of information. I want to think about it. I want to speak to my family doctor, I want to check with my pharmacist or therapist, I want to look on the Internet. I'll get back to you in a week or a year." You get back to me when you get back to me. It's not like you'll call me three months from now and I'll tell you that I won't see you because you didn't take me up on my gracious offer. People have to come to ADD treatment when they are ready to participate in it.

When that happens, you are welcome to bring your support person to the session, whether that's a parent, spouse, significant other, friend, or sibling, because you'll be hearing a lot of information and since we benefit from collateral observation of others, those who care about you may as well be informed at the same time.

The work that I do here is heavily results-based. You should expect a significant improvement. If all you get is a miserable little result, you shouldn't take the medication and I shouldn't prescribe it for you.

At the same time, it is hugely important for you to be accurate. Never come to my office and tell me what you hope will happen or what you think is what I want to hear or the exercise will be a colossal waste of your time and mine. And I am not in the business of wasting time. Just be accurate and I, in turn, will do my best to be accurate with you.

We are aiming for, and I am expecting, a significant improvement clinically. It would be to my advantage to say to you the opposite, that yours is a very complex case, and it will take all of my clinical skills and experience to see if we can get any result whatsoever. That is clearly not my agenda. Your presentation here, unique to you as it is, represents a very straightforward case of Attention Deficit Disorder. And if we approach it properly, with our oars in the water at the same time, we should achieve a great result.

You, like most of my patients, are not "missing parts". If you were, I would tell you. However, it is likely that you, like most of my patients, will need more than one stage of treatment. If you do need the second stage, don't be discouraged. This is not a character test. The medications are very helpful but all they are doing is allowing your healthy brain the opportunity to operate the way it is capable of. The medications don't make you nicer, smarter, or better. They just allow you to function the way you are fully able to.

Now we make an appointment for next week, where we will have an education session and I will lay out the treatment model for Attention Deficit Disorder, which you must remember is a fully treatable function problem as opposed to an illness. Here we go.

CHAPTER 11

How do we learn what we need to know?

Now that we've determined that you are a patient that needs both sides of the ADD coin treated, it's time for an Education Session. Here again, I will speak directly to you as my patient so that you can get the full understanding of the conceptual model and how it affects you physiologically.

Here we are in my private consultation office. There are not a lot of distractions so I can set my "screen" as it were (hands spread open beside my knees) down here. Now, let's say I get really hungry. I could just take this meeting over lunch in the middle of a busy restaurant. I could do just as good a job teaching there as I can here. All it would require is moving my screen from here (beside my knees) up to here (beside my eyes). You, on the other hand, can't make that move so easily. When you try to move your screen up to your eyes, it gets stuck. That's because there is a higher level of distractions, whether internal or external, that prevents you from bringing your full capacity to bear on an issue and attend to the task at hand.

So let's stay here in my office. I've got work to do. I have to be nimble in my thinking and edit on the fly. I have to be properly attentive, using focus and concentration, and be able to screen out distractions, both external and internal. I have to be appropriately inhibited to my circumstances, which is a fancy way of saying that I have to be properly behaved. I have to start at A, go on to B, C, D, digress for a bit, get to E, F, G, and digress a few times again on my way to Z. I have to do my duties along the way and I have to do a good job.

In order to achieve all of the work that gets me through the day, I have to depend on the outer two inches of my brain, the cortex, to be fast and rhythmic, metabolically-speaking (my hands are now flapping beside my head). By being fast and rhythmic, I can get a lot done.

Now let's say I am under great personal strain and before having this meeting, I just need to nip out to the corner bar and have five stiff drinks first. If that were the case, then my brain process would be quite different. Maybe I'd start at A and get to B but that would be about all. I'd get tangential; I'd be easily distracted. I'd get up out of my chair and wander around. I'd be inappropriately disinhibited because I'd be drunk. I'd make rude and inappropriate remarks. I'd be unable to do a good job. And I'd make an ass of myself all because of the difference between my cortex being fast and rhythmic (hands flapping in a coordinated rhythmic beat) and my cortex being slow and dysrhythmic (my hands now slowed down and out of sync).

There is some similarity here between me being drunk and you having ADD symptoms. Unlike mine, your whole cortex isn't affected (my hands sweeping around my head) but there is that certain small but significant part of your cortex that is stuck in a slow and dysrhythmic mode, that is never getting up and running.

Why is that? Here is the cortex (pointing to the outer two inches of the brain). Here are the billions of neurons and connections that make up your brain (my hands indicating the neurons descending from the cortex toward the base of the brain). Here is the brainstem (my hands compressed into a fist). Here is the spinal cord (my other hand indicating the tube of the spinal cord descending from the brain stem). That, in a simplified visual, is your central nervous system.

This is how it works. There is a beeping mechanism that sends out signals from the brainstem (my fist with the other hand regularly tapping out signals) up through the brain substance (my hands floating upwards and outwards from the brainstem) to the cortex to get the cortex up and running (my hands flapping rhythmically).

People with Attention Deficit Disorder do have a functioning brainstem (my hands indicating the rhythmic tapping of signals from the brain stem/fist). It sends out signals properly. But on their way to these small but important parts of the cortex, the signals get blocked or side-tracked (my hands indicating the signals being cut off).

What do we do about this? We use a mild stimulant. At this point, my patient would likely stop me with, "Dr. Hoffer, maybe you've forgotten the history. I'm having trouble as it is paying attention to things. Why would you give me a stimulant? I'll become more hyper, agitated, talking faster, and wacky? That's about the last thing I need. Why would you do that?"

Why I would do that, and why I'm going over this conceptual model with you is as follows. You swallow the stimulant. Fifteen minutes later, the stimulant starts to arrive at the brainstem. Now instead of sending out its regular signal (my hand tapping at a regular pace), the brainstem starts to send out harder, faster, stronger, and more frequent signals (my hand tapping out faster signals now). Some of these signals will still get blocked and side-tracked, but, because there are more of them, like water over the top of a dam, these signals now get around, under, over, and on through the blockages, reaching these important areas of the brain, allowing them to get up and running. As a result, you get the "paradoxical" response, the opposite intended of becoming more hyper/agitated/wacky. Instead, you become more focused, organized and able to maintain and sustain concentration for long periods of time. And that, in a nutshell, is what I call the "Stage I" mild stimulant treatment for Attention Deficit Disorder, which also implies that there is more than one stage to the treatment.

There are two types of stimulants we can choose from and both are excellent, safe options. One is Ritalin (methylphenidate) and the other, Dexedrine. They come in two formats that matter for our purpose. One is a 4-hour tablet, taken after breakfast, after lunch, and taken in the afternoon, approximately 4 hours apart. The other is a once-daily long-acting format, which lasts about the same length of time. Taking the pill once a day means generally less side effects because there is less fluctuation of the blood level. Although the long-acting stimulant may be preferable, I don't usually start with it because if it fails to work for you, it fails for 12 hours instead of 4. Also, the short-acting tablets are easier to ramp up to a standard dose for size and age and easier to make the switch later to the equivalent long-acting dose.

With respect to side effects, let's look at three categories: immediate, medium-term, and long-term. Immediate side effects appear in the first few days, the most important of which answers this question: Are you getting more hyper and agitated rather than getting more focused and concentrated? With your history, it is highly unlikely for you to become agitated but it's something to watch for.

The medium-term side effects mainly occur within the first 2-3 weeks of starting the dose. These include diminished appetite, delayed onset of sleep, dry mouth, jaw clenching, eye twitches, shoulder shrugs, mild headache, and feeling your heart is beating a little faster for a few moments in the day. These are generally minor and tend to quickly ameliorate within the first few weeks so they are essentially physiologically insignificant.

Long-term side effects implies that the medication is working and that is why you are taking it long term. Therefore, if the medication is working, that means there are generally no long-term side effects.

As discussed in the previous chapter, once patients are sufficiently educated to make the decision to go ahead with treatment, I give them a prescription and an agenda that takes them to a standard dose for size and age over the course of the first 7-8 days (see Table I). We need one week to see if it works, two weeks to "tailor" the dose—a little higher here, a little lower there—and then another two weeks to run with the tailored dose (or switch to the long-acting format). We meet regularly during that time.

At the end of 4-5 weeks, patients return for a major review session, at which point I ask how they are doing. One-quarter of people come back and say some version of the following. "Oh my God, you are the greatest doctor ever. I am so much more focused. I'm more organized. I'm getting more done. I'm doing better at home and work and/or school. Maybe a little tough in the morning before the medication has kicked in, maybe a little tough in the evening when the medication is wearing off. I can deal with that. You are the greatest."

The other three-quarters of my patients come back for the review session and give me a variation on this theme. "Look Dr. Hoffer, I am more focused on things. I guess that's good. But I am really disappointed and underwhelmed. I thought this was going to make a big difference in my life. But I'm still sticky, I'm still stubborn, I still make all sorts of excuses as to why I'm not getting things done on time. I still don't read social cues well. My time management sucks. I don't prioritize well. I still procrastinate all the time. I'm not motivated like I should be. Like I said, I'm really disappointed."

At this point I make the joke that there are two diagnostic categories at play here. In the first quarter of my patients, where I am the greatest doctor alive, the diagnostic category is that Dr. Hoffer is really smart. In the rest of my patients, the diagnostic category is that I am really a jerk. How does one make sense of this dichotomy? The fact is, every patient I see falls into one of these two categories, regardless of their socioeconomic, racial, ethnic, or religious background. How does one conceptualize this phenomenon?

By now, you've probably heard about people being described as either left-brained or right-brained. How does that description of thinking impact our understanding of the duality when it comes to treatment for ADD?

The stereotype of the left-brained person is that of the accountant who can focus and concentrate on tiny details in the middle of a hurricane for hours but who may be a little colorless or humorless in his social life. As it turns out, that side of the brain is heavily influenced by the dopamine neurotransmitter.

On the other hand, the stereotype of the right-brained person is that of the creative artist. These people have right-brained attributes that are mainly norepinephrine mediated and will likely answer yes to the following questions about themselves:

- Can you delay gratification when you have to?
- Can you find and hit your own pause button on your personal control panel so when faced with a decision, rather than just blurting something out or impulsively avoiding it, you can pause, think things through, weigh consequences, and then decide, all in microseconds?
- Are you aware of how you come across to others?
- Are you sensitive to other people's perceptions of you?
- Can you be a team player when necessary?
- Can you be flexible and have a sense of humour, particularly under stress?
- Can you pick up on social cues and social nuance?
- Can you time manage properly?
- Can you prioritize effectively?
- Can you be motivated when you need to be?
- Can you avoid procrastinating to your own detriment?

We are all, more or less, a combination of left and right brainedness. So when patients return for their 4-5 week review session, and they tell me that they are doing great and how wonderful I am, I refer to them as having what I would call "left-brained ADD". The process of the stimulant sending out signals from the brainstem, up through the brain substance to the cortex is happening on the "left" side or dopamine-mediated side of the brain. You give these people a dopamine-mediated medication like one of the stimulants (Ritalin or Dexedrine) and "voila", you get a great treatment result.

But in three-quarters of my cases, and most likely you, the problem of the signals coming from the brainstem up through the brain substance to the cortex is happening on *both* sides of the brain, including on the norepinephrine–mediated side of the equation. And in order to get that side of the brain up and running, I usually will need to add in a norepinephrine-impacting antidepressant.

Now most people will stop me here and say, "But Dr. Hoffer, I'm not depressed. Why would you give me an antidepressant?"

To combat depression in adults, an antidepressant takes about 3-4 weeks to start helping and often 6-10 weeks to fully kick in. For treating ADD, however, if this medication works, we see improvement within 7-10 days, sometimes as early as day 5. Why is that? Because it is not working on an antidepressant basis; it is working on a "pause button" or "anti-impulse" basis.

The classic story I tell is of the teenage boy, already on a stimulant medication to help him with his focus and concentration, coming home from school. He is greeted at the door by his mother.

"Hi honey, how was your day?"

"Fine," the boy replies.

"Do you have any homework?"

"No, Mom, I don't have any homework."

The next day, the mother gets a phone call or e-mail from the school. Her son hasn't handed in his latest book report and assignments, and he hasn't completed his homework. The mother thinks: "My kid is a liar and he's lazy."

So what happened? When the mother asked her son if he had any homework, the following occurred in the young fellow's brain: "I have a lot of homework, I hate homework. No, Mom, I don't have any homework." No pause button, no weighing of consequences or consideration of options. Just immediate impulsive avoidance.

When we add the Stage II treatment to the Stage I treatment and it works, the scenario unfolds differently.

"Hi honey, how was your day?"

"Fine."

"Do you have any homework?"

"Yes, I've got quite a bit of homework. I'm going to head to my room soon and get started on it."

The teenager goes to do his homework. The mom is thrilled and shocked.

Now what has happened? The response starts out the same way in the teenager's brain but then it takes a turn. "I've got a lot of homework. I hate homework. *But* (here is the boy hitting the pause button that was not previously accessible) I'm doing way better in school. My teachers are off my back. My marks are way up. My parents are pleased. That little jerk in class who's always saying "Whatcha get?" after each math test is going to get a shock when I turn to him next time and say, "I got an A, what did you get?" Okay,

I'm going to do my homework." And this happens in microseconds. In other words, the pace of the conversation is identical in both scenarios.

What are some of the questions that patients ask me about these medications? The most frequent one is "Can I get addicted to this?" You get addicted to something that gives you a buzz or a kick or a high. What we are talking about here is the opposite of that high feeling and in fact, the medication protects an ADD person from developing drug and alcohol problems. When the drug works, you become more successful. You become more capable and more confident. You are less likely to feel frustrated and marginalized. You are less likely to hang out with other marginalized people looking for alternative solutions to help them feel better, such as alcohol or drugs.

People also ask: "Let's say this works. Do I have to take it every day?" The answer is no. These medications that we will be starting with, the stimulant medications, work only for the 4, 8, or 12 hours that they last each day. The medication works only for that quantum of time that is taken for. If you take it on a Monday and a Tuesday, skip it on Wednesday, and take it Thursday, it only works on the day you take it. So some people will take it Monday through Friday for work/school purposes, then skip it on the Saturday when they sleep late and run some errands, but then take it on Sunday to help with organization and paperwork. As a result, there is some flexibility in using the Stage I stimulant treatment. That said, most people, doing well on a stimulant, want to take it every day because they like doing well and they enjoy being able to focus and sustain that concentration throughout the day.

However, if we move on to the Stage II treatment, and it works, that medication must be taken on a daily basis for it to work properly. Like most medications, this one works on a "constant level" basis. So, if one day, you skip the Stage I stimulant treatment, you should still continue the Stage II treatment that day.

Patients also ask how long they will be on the medication? My standard answer is that approximately 60% of patients who have ADD symptoms in childhood will continue to have these problems persist into adulthood. About 40% will "outgrow" their symptoms by their mid-20's. We don't know which group you will end up in. So my recommendation is that we reassess all the way along but, for academic purposes, you will likely continue to need treatment through your undergraduate period at college or university, which captures both the time frame (early to mid-20's) and the prognosis. The good news is that most ADD people, once they get treated, go on to do what other smart capable people go on to do.

For those people who don't "outgrow" their treatment, they will end up needing and benefitting from it for many years. However, approximately half of my adult patients who need Stage II treatment will, after 12-18 months, be able to stop the second medication and still experience improved motivation and diminished procrastination issues. It is almost like they are able, through that period, to have inculcated and ingrained more successful habits. Or maybe they have been able to "grow" a connection to their own pause button during that time, enabling them to stop, think things through, and then make better and more successful decisions.

People come to see me. I educate them. If they decide to go ahead, we go through the process as outlined. Everything we do is based on the results. These first two stages of treatment represent what I would refer to as "the heavy lifting done." There may be refinements to the treatment but what I've covered today is 85-90% of what you'll likely need.

People go through this process. If it works, they come back and say something like following. "Dr. Hoffer, when I first came to see you, I was hopeful you could help me. But I was also skeptical. After all, I've been this way a long time. What is the likelihood anything will improve all that much? And I wasn't keen on all this medication. I didn't want to be hyped up on this or hopped up on that. And, frankly, you seemed much too sure of yourself. That was a little off-putting. But now that I've been through this process, I am operating at the best level I've ever functioned at, the level that I want to keep functioning at. In addition, I am much more composed; I am much more in control of my decision-making and myself. I finally feel that I have my hands on my own steering wheel rather than feeling I am always like a pinball bouncing off the bumpers of life. And it feels utterly natural, like this is me finally getting a chance to be who I really am."

Again, these words emphasize that Attention Deficit Disorder is not an illness but rather is a functional problem. You don't get that kind of result treating illness; you get that kind of result correcting a function problem.

And that concludes our education session.

TABLE I - Short-Acting Stimulant Trial Period

Ritalin 10 mg tabs **OR** Dexedrine 5 mg tabs

	After Breakfast (8 am)	After lunch (12 noon)	Late Afternoon (4:15 pm)
Day #			
(1)	1 (tablet)	—	—
(2)	1	1	—
(3)	1	1	—

(Call Dr. Hoffer to report / decide on dose)

Then if ok:

(4)	1	1	1
(5)	1 ½	1	1
(6)	1 ½	1 ½	1

(Call again/report again)

Then if ok:

(7)	1 ½	1 ½	1
(8)	1 ½ (or 2)	1 ½	1

(Meet for an appointment)

CHAPTER 12

What happens at the next two appointments?

After the education session, some of my patients (perhaps 20%) decide not to commence treatment immediately. They want time to mull over what I have said, speak to their family doctor and/or consult with their therapist. Some will want to read up on the subject either in books or on the Internet. A few will want to check with their pharmacist.

The majority of patients I meet with are ready to commence treatment right away. By the time they enter my office, most have struggled with the vagaries of life for a long time and are keen to experience an end to their frustration and suffering. They are looking forward to the opportunity for a transformative clinical response. Of those patients, most will be given a prescription for one of the Stage I stimulants (Ritalin or Dexedrine) along with an accompanying agenda (Table I in the preceding chapter). The patient will have spoken with me a couple of times during the 7-8 ensuing days to ensure that they are on the right track and to be able to alert me if they are experiencing any excessive untoward side effects.

Dexedrine and Ritalin are the two safest, most effective therapeutic options in the stimulant category. Though similar, they are not identical. Many patients will respond to both medications but a significant proportion will respond to one and not the other or will respond significantly better to one than the other. It is very important to ascertain the "best fit" for each patient. In a remarkable stroke of good fortune, the overwhelming majority of patients in my clinical experience will clearly respond to one of these two medications, even if they haven't responded to the initial choice of stimulant.

Both medications have their advantages. Ritalin has the capacity to provide a stronger "heavier" focus quality in some patients. Consistent with my treatment model, that is because Ritalin represents a pure "dopamine" play; it works on the "left-brained" focus and concentration part of the brain's function. Some people, particularly, teens and young adults, may find themselves noting that they don't like the impact of the Ritalin, which can have them feeling less outgoing, less social, and less personable. This effect, seen most often when the dose is being adjusted upwards, is due to the dopamine-centric nature of Ritalin. It provides more focus, more organization, better attention to detail but all at the expense of being less tuned in socially.

Dexedrine works mainly on the dopamine neurotransmitter but works a little bit on the "other side of the coin", the norepinephrine neurotransmitter. Because of this better and slightly more balanced impact, adult patients in particular tend to favour using Dexedrine (either short-acting tablets taken 3 times a day or long-acting Vyvanse once daily). When Dexedrine is preferred, the patient will almost always note that the experience feels smoother and does not negatively impact personality issues. In my practice, Dexedrine is probably used 55-60% of the time while Ritalin is used 40-45% of the time.

When the patient returns for the first session after treatment with a stimulant has been initiated, usually 7-8 days after the education session, I am interested to hear about the experience. I first ask about side effects and whether those side effects have already started to lessen in severity. Dry mouth, feeling a little nervous, some trouble falling asleep at night, experiencing some increase in heart rate for a few moments during the day, and diminished appetite are often noted as worse in the first few days and are already diminishing by the time we meet.

Next, I inquire as to the "effect" (or benefit) the patient feels. The majority of properly diagnosed patients will begin to itemize a series of significant improvements they have seen in just a few days. Better ability to focus and concentrate for longer periods is the key improvement I am looking for. Increased reading, improved diligence in sticking to a task, and being more organized are other effects that are frequently noted. Many patients note that they feel their brain has finally "woken up" and they have more energy to usefully deploy in the service of their obligations. This observation is not due to them being "stimulated" or "hyper" but rather is due to the medication facilitating the "reversal" of the under-aroused state of the parts of the cerebral cortex responsible for the ADD symptoms.

Most patients are delighted by this initial, quite remarkable, change. They also find it somewhat hard to believe. Many are reluctant to express their underlying fear that this profound improvement might be just a temporary change that will soon fade. Others express bitterness and question why they have never been given this opportunity before despite having struggled so hard for so long.

After letting the patient know that it may be too early to tell, I ask about how any procrastination and motivation problems may have changed. I want my patients to be thinking about the "two sides of the coin" right from the get-go. A number of patients will say that it is that it is too soon to know but some will exclaim that they are getting down to things that they have constantly been putting off and delaying—doing their taxes, cleaning their room, organizing their desk, or whatever else needs doing. I tell them that they will get tired of me asking them at each follow-up appointment about attention/ focus/ concentration and procrastination/ motivation/ time management.

As long as the direction of treatment is promising, I continue tailoring the medication upwards. One exception is the patient who is more focused but having a quantum of side effects that are unpleasant and hard to endure. In such a case, I wait an extra week or two while the body "acclimates" to the presence of stimulant medication. The other exception is the patient who feels the dose is already just right, in which case it remains unchanged for another week after which time the patient will report in. Often, the patient will call and say that perhaps they might want to adjust their dose then.

"Tailoring a dose" of stimulant is a very straightforward process. After the first 7-8 days, my general practice is to increase the dose by ½ tablet increments every couple of days. A typical agenda looks like this:

	8 a.m.	12 noon	4:15 p.m.
Monday	1 ½	1	1
Tuesday	1 ½	1 ½	1
Wednesday	1 ½	1 ½	1
Thursday	1 ½	1 ½	1 ½
Then if OK			
Friday	1 ½	1 ½	1 ½
Saturday	1 ½	1 ½	1 ½
Sunday	2	1 ½	1 ½
Monday	2	1 ½	1 ½
Then call to report (or meet for an appointment)			

I explain to my patients that the tailoring process looks at the balance between effect (benefit) and side effect. If we increase the dose and you have the same levels of benefit and side effect, that's a losing proposition. Why take more medication to get the same result? Or if we increase the dose and get the same level of benefit but even more side effects, that is also a losing proposition. With an increased dose, there is often a slight increase initially in side effect, which usually settles within a few days. What we are looking for, ideally, is improved benefit versus relatively minimal side effect. That is called the enhanced "therapeutic ratio".

What if the patient returns post-treatment and reports no benefit and an absence of significant side effects? Surprisingly, this is not a common occurrence. In this case, I will probe further to ensure that the patient did not in fact see signs of sharper focus. If the patient then acknowledges some modest improvement, I will explain we should continue the tailoring process until we obtain a more robust response as we achieve a better dose/response level.

However, some patients clearly do not have a decent response or any response at all for that matter. It is still very important to inquire about the presence of side effects. What you do not want is the rare case where someone reports feeling too agitated or "hyped up" on the medication. Keep in mind that feeling "a bit nervous" or "jittery" in the first few days is a much different side effect than agitation. If the side effects are minimal, even without benefit, the next step is clear. I tell the patient that these are early days and that it is very important to establish the right fit for Stage I treatment. I then prescribe the other stimulant (Ritalin if I started with Dexedrine; Dexedrine if I started with Ritalin) and give the same starting agenda for the new stimulant. The patient is instructed to call me by day 2-3 and again at day 4-5 with a follow-up appointment in a week's time.

Fortuitously, properly diagnosed ADD patients will almost always respond to one or the other of the two stimulant families. In old medical literature, the rate of non-response was quoted as high as 30% of patients. My own experience would lower that number to less than 5%.

The exceptions to this rule fall roughly into three categories. One category is obvious. There are some people who are acutely sensitive to stimulant medication and cannot tolerate the side effects. They become nervous and "turn green" with nausea. The second group are patients for whom the medication simply does not work.

The third group is more interesting. This is the cohort of patients who clearly have ADD symptomatology and, when I initiate a trial of stimulant medication expecting a robust Stage I response, I see instead a distinctly muted one. "A little better focus, maybe" is how the patient describes feeling. After switching to the alternative stimulant, expecting a stronger showing, I receive the same "meh" response — "about the same as the first medication you had me on." How is this response happening? We see that these people have feathers, webbed feet, waddle, and quack. How can they not be a duck?

What I now understand is that this group — often composed of adult men between 35-60 years of age — represents an entity where the Stage I treatment is subdued by the massive interference that their executive dysfunction represents. Their brain literally can't allow the stimulant treatment to work properly because they are so "self-dysregulated" with an overabundance of impulsivity and a severe motivational deficiency that the stimulant can't operate properly in the brain. What I do with these patients is I ask them to tell which of the two stimulant treatments is the one they felt best on, even if the improvement was modest. I then proceed with the stimulant Stage I treatment and begin the executive function Stage II treatment. Within 7-14 days, if it works, both sides of the coin start to become engaged in both better attention and greater executive function and productivity. It is almost like the Stage II issues represent an "overhang" preventing the "rise" of the Stage I attentional improvement. Once the Stage II improvement commences, the overhang is removed and both sides of the coin become operative and engaged.

Fortunately, most of my patients respond with a very clear improvement in their capacity to sustain focus and concentration, even if they still have challenges with procrastination/motivation issues. As the dose is tailored upwards, the process of refining the therapeutic response is important so as to achieve the best possible result. There are two main reasons for this outcome. The first is obvious: the better able a person is to effectively maintain and deploy focus, the more capable and successful they will be in achieving their goals.

The second reason is less obvious but also very important in the understanding of the treatment model. Though I have written conceptually, the second stage treatment is very much contingent on the presence of the first stage (stimulant) treatment. It is much more accurate to conceptualize the treatment not as "side-by-side" but as the second stage treatment working off the platform that the first stage treatment has created. Like the foundations of a house, it is necessary to build a solid base. Without that base, subsequent treatment stages are essentially rendered ineffectual.

Most patients I see are delighted and relieved when they experience initial improvements in daily function. Many will talk about the switch finally being turned on, the curtain lifting, and their brain awakening. As they start to do better, one of the questions I am frequently asked is "How long will it take for me to rebuild my lost confidence?". It doesn't matter if you are 14 years old of 54 years old. The time frame is essentially the same and the good news is that it doesn't take 14 or 54 more years.

I review with my patients the three phases of the recovery and repair of one's confidence. The first phase happens during the first month of treatment. You see something a positive result and you feel excited and hopeful. You are able to get more done, read more, and achieve with facility. You feel you are on your way and this must be the answer. And that feeling, that you are finally on the right track, reminds you there have been other times in your life when you felt that you were on the right track and your hopes ended in bitter disappointment. So you tell yourself that although it appears that something good has started, you don't know if this isn't just a trick that fades. You are wary, and for good reason.

The second phase of confidence recovery happens in the next two months. During that time, you are starting to do better on a dependable day-by-day basis. By the end of this phase, you see that you are able to do just as well as the people you used to consider "regular effective people" who you wished you were more like. Now you are operating not just better than you used to but just as well as those you wanted to emulate.

The third and final phase occurs in the fourth month of treatment. It is the last phase of the process of rebuilding one's confidence. During this period, this phrase resonates: "It doesn't matter what they throw down on the table any day because you can eat right through it."

For a minority of my patients, perhaps 20%, Stage I treatment is all they need. These patients have functional dopamine inefficiency in their neurophysiologic transmission and the introduction of the stimulant medication corrects the functional issue. For most of my patients, however, Stage I is just the beginning. Now, they are ready to move on to the second stage of treatment, which I will outline in the following chapter.

To conclude this chapter, I have selected as an example a recent patient's initial personal history (in his own words) followed by his experience of Stage I treatment, which was, in his case, sufficient to help him live to his fullest capabilities.

Patient's Personal History

It's 10:16 pm on the night before my appointment and my girlfriend finally pushed me to get this done, since she knows how important it is for both of us!

Ever since elementary school, I remember being restless, unable to focus for the duration of the entire lesson, drifting away thinking of stuff I would love to be doing instead. This led to teachers labeling me as one with "great potential, but lazy." Ever since I was young, I would believe that doing things my way on my own time was vastly superior to predefined methods of accomplishing or achieving things. I would get bored easily, looking for excitement elsewhere, unmotivated to do anything I am not truly passionate about, while spending hours and even days focused on things that were exciting me at the time.

As an adult, I feel that a lot of these issues still exist and as I study ADD and ADHD more closely, I am both terrified and relieved. I now have a better understanding of why I went through three different employers in 2015 and ended up on Employment Insurance while trying to do freelance work. After I was laid off in November of 2015, I felt useless and fell into depression. I started taking Cipralex to bring my emotional state back to normal, which I am glad to say is helping a lot.

Dealing with freelance work, though, is very difficult, since I tend to only talk to potential and existing clients when I am in a good mood and excited. After the contract is signed, I tend to feel like I've accomplished enough and can reward myself with a bit of leisure/distraction that ends up being days instead of minutes. I set up a schedule to wake up early and get on my computer to do work but despite all the tools and resources being right in front of me, I find myself reading/watching stuff that although is very interesting and exciting, has nothing to do with my current assignment. More stuff piles up as the days go by and then in the state of utter panic and adrenaline rushes (often after staying up the whole night procrastinating), I start trying to pull off the impossible. It is surprising how much I can accomplish under pressure in such short periods of time, but I would be living a much calmer and happier life if I actually didn't put things off until the last moment. I believe I would still be happy, employed with more money and more reasons to wake up and be energetic every morning!

The other state I can find myself in is hyper-focus for even an entire weekend, where I ignore food, sleep and basically anything else. I am only in this state when I am working on my own exciting projects that require me to really push myself in the areas I really enjoy working in, including programming, designing user interfaces and user experiences, especially when related to video gaming. As far as I can remember, I relied on the help of caffeine—at first using just coffee, then energy drinks, and now sticking to 200 mg caffeine tablets to eliminate all the sugar, etc. in drinks. I find it much easier to get started in the morning if I take one or two 200 mg tablets 20-30 minutes before my actual alarm clock time (I wake up to take the pills and go back to bed for 20-30 minutes).

Another habit/trend I notice that seems to be consistent with other ADHD symptoms is impulsive spending, which in conjunction with my poor work ethic has led to many difficult financial situations. My credit rating has been destroyed by my frivolous spending and although I am on the path to recovery and most dues are paid, the damage is going to take a long time to fix. Another thing that I realized that is not normal in all people is the ability to remember things from years (even just few) ago. If you were to ask me what I did between 2008 and 2013, I would have to go back to my e-mails to put together scraps of memories. I don't remember many things I notice others do remember like what they did in the summer of 2012, etc. For me, it's just blank.

Patient's Update

It's been roughly one month since I first saw Dr. Hoffer, but it really feels like an eternity has passed. My first visit was quite quick, but incredibly informative. I had a chance to confirm many assumptions I've made over the years regarding WHY things are happening the way they are, or rather, why they weren't happening the way I always wanted them to.

The past month was incredibly informative. Ever since the first visit, which resulted in a lot of new knowledge and an adequate medication plan, I feel like not only am I finally back to "normal", but I have actually exceeded the wildest expectations that I, and probably even Dr. Hoffer, had.

As I am typing this letter at 11:30 am on a Thursday, starting my day with a hearty breakfast, a walk and a few errands around the area (this morning's to-do list would've taken a week just a few months ago), I am realizing how much has actually changed. I was wondering how to structure this "post mortem" and I think it's best to give a quick list of things I am most proud of!

First, in the past month, I've spent 25 minutes total playing video games, and that was on the first day of treatment. My time perception has drastically changed. No longer am I content with "right here, right now" as I always used to be. This newly found love for the "future me" led me to getting my finances in order, reviewing my credit report and ensuring all of the outstanding matters are resolved, opening a savings account and actually making more money on my own (web development contracting) than I ever have before. My days are much more structured, I maintain daily, weekly, monthly and "far into the future" lists of tasks and I get through even the toughest tasks with ease.

Second, things that I used to do as a distraction or my favourite form of procrastination just ceased to exist. I finally learned the true value of time and how persistence, determination and hard work is not only rewarding but very liberating. I have to admit, I still tend to procrastinate here and there, but this is a new form of hyper-productive procrastination. In the past month, I've managed to learn, understand and feel comfortable using a plethora of programming concepts, project management tactics and marketing strategies. Each moment I drift away from things I have to do is spent on actually learning how can I do things better the moment I return to the task at hand. It is an incredible feeling that has brought many benefits beyond my professional life—being happy and proud of my work and newly created lifestyle heavily influences and encourages those around me to strive for the best.

Last but not least, I am in total control of my life. In the past, I would tend to spend more time and energy going around problems than trying to solve them. Today, I have no problems. I just have a list of tasks with varied levels of difficulty, but I am ready to tackle them head on. No issue or challenge is bigger than me anymore. In fact, my eagerness to tackle life's struggle is directly proportional to the complexity and difficulty of that struggle. I feel happy, satisfied, with my daily life, focused on the near and far future and in total control of "my universe". The feeling of euphoria that used to knock on my door once in a blue moon is with me at all times now. By the time I go to sleep each evening, I am just ecstatic to start the next day because today, I finally know the value of small steps toward big goals.

Dr. Hoffer and his "no bullshit" method of dealing with dysfunctional brains and disconnected minds gave me the best gift I never even knew was obtainable: the gift of living up to the potential I knew was there, but for years remained a dream out of reach. For that, I will be forever grateful.

CHAPTER 13

What is The Stage II Treatment all about?

In the preceding chapter, the Stage I treatment for Attention Deficit Disorder was profiled. For many physicians, the use of a psychostimulant for the patient diagnosed with ADD is both the beginning and the end of the treatment effort. If the patient responds to the medication and the inadequate capacity to pay attention is enhanced then isn't that the goal of treatment? After all, the "attention" of the "Attention" Deficit Disorder has been improved on. Case closed, right?

Not at all. However, if the doctor's belief system dictates that the problem has been treated and whatever else is left is a separate issue, then no further treatment effort will be considered. In particular, if the patient returns and says something like "I'm still not getting my act together" or "I'm still having a hell of a time getting started on important projects," they are likely to be told something wise and useless like "You'll just have to try harder," or "You have to learn to establish your priorities," or even "You have to stop being so lazy."

In my office, I am very specific with patients. They are instructed to look out for not just for the improvement in their focus/concentration/attention but also for their procrastination/motivation/time management/prioritization. I consider it "half a loaf" (at best) if someone returns to my office in the subsequent few weeks with better capacity to pay attention and no improvement in their overall "executive functionality".

What do other doctors do at this juncture? Often, the stimulant dose will be increased in an effort to achieve a "fuller" result. As mentioned earlier, once a stimulant dose has been properly tailored and adjusted, giving more is of little value and runs the risk of creating noxious side effects for the patient (nausea, agitation, and irritability). Increasing the dopamine won't generally increase the norepinephrine side of the coin because the fact is, you can't get to here (norepinephrine) from there (dopamine).

Sometimes the doctor may suggest talk therapy. This route is generally doomed to failure. It fails not because psychotherapy is useless; psychotherapy is an enormously effective treatment for many psychiatric difficulties. It fails because psychotherapy can't address the self-regulatory challenges of the ADD person any more than squinting and eating more carrots can address the optometric challenges of the person who needs glasses.

Sometimes the more enlightened physician will refer the patient to a life coach or ADD coach but doing so at this stage may be premature. An experienced ADD coach can be very instrumental in helping a person define the challenges they face and establish parameters on how to address them. But they still can't address the infuriating and frustrating tendency for ADD people to react impulsively due to their lack of access to their own personal "pause button". ADD coaches can be enormously helpful, though, once Stage II issues are actually treated properly.

After the first few weeks of the Stage I treatment effort, my patients return for a review session. The distinct minority of my patients are "all better" at that point. They are doing remarkably well on "both sides of the coin". They are able to concentrate more efficiently and for sustained periods of time. They are much less easily distracted by extraneous stimuli. They are also much more competent and efficient. They are no longer procrastinating to their detriment. They are able to get things accomplished and to start, continue, and complete.

What do all the rest report? Without exception, the theme I hear over and over is the inability to achieve a state of self-regulatory diligence. "I'm more focused but I still procrastinate all the time. I still say the wrong thing at the wrong time. I can't initiate the tasks I have to do. I'm not bad when I finally get started on things but getting started is such an overwhelming problem in itself. I still feel so impulsive. I still leave things to the last minute. I am still so disorganized."

At that point in the treatment process, usually 4-5 weeks in, I will initiate a discussion about Stage II treatment. If the patient is generally positive about their improvement and their executive function issues are somewhat improved, I will usually wait another few weeks before considering the initiation of the second stage. For some people, the initial "honeymoon stage" of improvement is strong enough to last 8-12 weeks. But for most, there is not a full and robust response to the Stage I effort. I begin the discussion about the need to address all of the "self-regulation dysfunction issues" now.

The first point I make is a restatement: this is not a character test. I tell my patients that having difficulty with procrastination/motivation issues is absolutely part and parcel of having ADD. So much so that, in fact, when a person provides a clear initial history to me of both attentional and executive function symptomatology, I am actually surprised if they return for the review session following the Stage I treatment and tell me they are all better. If a person returns with improved attention but still is bedeviled by their glaring defects in their adult capacities, that is not evidence of their adult unworthiness or inferiority. It is merely that we have so far only addressed one side of the coin.

The second point that I make is that the second medication works synergistically in conjunction with the first (stimulant) medication. Essentially, I describe it as the second medication working off the platform that the first medication creates. This building block analogy explains why the likelihood of success is so much greater than just trying the second stage treatment by itself.

For the rest of the discussion about Stage II treatment, I'll return now to the role of doctor, speaking directly to you the patient in my office, and I'll provide you with the information you require to make an educated decision about the second stage of the treatment. (Note that this is the discussion I reserve for young adult and adult patients; the discussion with children and younger teens is similar but different.)

The medication we are going to add to your current stimulant regimen is an antidepressant named Wellbutrin. Although marketed under a different name (Zyban), the exact same medication is used to help people stop smoking. I am not using it in your case as an antidepressant nor as a smoking cessation agent.

Wellbutrin works to enhance the transmission in the brain of the norepinephrine neurotransmitter. Unlike most antidepressants, which impact the serotonin neurotransmitter, Wellbutrin is different. And because it is different, it doesn't cause the usual serotonin-related side effects of nausea, fatigue, sexual dysfunction, and weight gain. Wellbutrin generally isn't associated with those side effects at all.

The majority of my patients on Wellbutrin, in combination with their stimulant treatment, experience very few side effects. I will go over the side effects with you but you are very likely not to experience any of them. The medication can initially lead to a feeling of some anxiety or "jitteriness"; this is usually transient. It is generally weight-neutral; some people will notice a diminution in their appetite. One in 200 will develop a red rash after the first week generally on the lower jaw, neck, and upper chest area, which usually will respond to an antihistamine. Occasionally, on hotter days, you may notice increased sweating. This is generally a minor side effect. You will notice on the pharmacy printout that this medication can potentially lower your seizure threshold. In the absence of a history of seizures, this is more of theoretical interest. In rare circumstances, a person can get agitated on this medication. Agitated doesn't mean "I'm a little nervous"; it means "I'm going to punch that policeman over there." That is a bad sign and you have to contact me if you feel that way and stop the medication. That said, most of the people on Wellbutrin notice few if any side effects.

Most of my adult patients start on 150 mg once a day in the morning for the first week (the long-acting once-daily XL formulation). Then you will report back to me. If there are no significant side effects, I will generally increase to 300 mg in the morning for the second week. If there are some side effects at the end of the first week, I will keep you on 150 mg for the second week and then decide on the dose for the third week. If you are going to see a benefit with this Stage II treatment, you will see it in these first 2-3 weeks. There is little benefit to be gained staying on this stage of treatment if you have not seen a benefit in that time frame.

What is the benefit we are looking for? Unlike an antidepressant effect, which generally would appear over a number of weeks, if this medication works properly, you will start to see a benefit within 7-10 days, sometimes as early as day 5.

Look out for the following improvements:

- Gee, I got so much done today. I started/continued/completed and then worked to start/continue/complete the next thing on my list. I never do that. Previously, if there was something that I needed to do, I'd go check the fridge, look at my e-mail, speak to a friend, and then start something unimportant which had nothing to do with what I needed to do.

- I felt like doing more. I got things done which I usually avoid. I was more diligent. I didn't procrastinate as much as I usually do. I felt more motivated. I didn't feel so tired and dragged out.

- I was more aware of what was going on around me in terms of social

cues. I had more of a pause button. I said the right thing at the right
time after I had quickly thought it through.

- *I was more organized. I was able to prioritize better. My time*
  management was much smoother.

- *I felt more composed. I wasn't as easily flustered or overwhelmed. I felt*
  like I had more self-control.

This understanding that the Stage I treatment is truly only
"half-a-loaf" for the majority of the ADD population is of critical
importance. It is like being very pleased that you can hit a forehand in
tennis really well but at the same time, you can't hit a decent
backhand. You never get a chance to become who you truly are
capable of becoming. This is why I often tell patients that once we
get both sides of the treatment engaged, the patient will finally get a
chance to really meet their true self for the first time. This game
changing experience is well demonstrated in the case that follows.

David struggled with feeling inferior all of his life because
of his undiagnosed and untreated ADD. When you meet David, you
see that he is clearly very intelligent, articulate, personable, and
ridiculously handsome. Yet he always experienced the palpable sense
that he was "faking his way through". As a mature student, he gained
access to medical school and came to see me after he had obtained
Stage I treatment, which had been partially helpful only.

In the following narrative written by David, take note of how
his story evolves once he gets the opportunity to have a successful
Stage II treatment as well. David has become fully successful, fully
confident, and fully realized. But this is who he is and always was.

What he never had before was the opportunity to meet his true self. This case demonstrates why it is so important for all ADD patients to understand what can be accomplished in addressing full functionality, not just the "attentional" aspect of the condition.

David's Personal Statement

During my second semester of medical school, it became very hard for me to focus and concentrate on both studying and paying attention in class. I would find myself either daydreaming in class or experiencing extreme fatigue when I fought the urge to daydream and instead tried to concentrate on the lesson. It was as if I had to summon sheer willpower just to focus, listen, take notes, and try to learn during class. This mental effort would translate into physical fatigue where I would find myself almost falling asleep in class. Later at night, the problem worsened because I would have to devote extra time to study to make up for not paying attention in class. I started to experience a great deal of anxiety surrounding studying because I was unable to focus, concentrate, or remember much of what I attempted to study. This anxiety then led to increased procrastination surrounding studying.

The second semester carried a much heavier course load compared to the first. My wife and daughter also came to live with me at this time (we were living in separate countries during first semester). The combination of an increased school workload and added family responsibilities proved too much. By the second set of block exams, I was failing every course. I felt overwhelmed because I was unable to focus, concentrate, remember/recall material, or organize my schedule so I could meet the demands of both medical school and spend adequate time with my wife and daughter. Meeting my breaking point, I took a leave of absence to avoid having failed courses on my transcripts. I also planned to transfer to another school where the class schedule facilitated more self study time.

During the leave of absence, we went to Brazil (my wife is from Brazil) and I sought help from a psychiatrist. She prescribed Ritalin and I could not believe the difference. I was able to focus, concentrate, and recall material. For the first time in my life, I found studying to be an enjoyable and relaxing experience. The anxiety and worry about not being able to focus and get work done was gone. I was able to use my time much more effectively than I ever had in my life. Studying was something I began to look forward to and not fear. The procrastination surrounding studying ended because I no longer found it stressful. In fact, one of the biggest improvements I experienced after starting medication was that I no longer worried about studying because I knew I was learning and getting my work done during the time I spent studying. Another benefit was the positive impact on my relationships with my wife and daughter. The constant worry and anxiety over not being able to focus, which would then trigger irritability and anger, had substantially reduced and I was able to be more present and patient with them.

Importantly, my marks also increased dramatically. I was on the Dean's list in all semesters afterwards except one, tutored courses in Pharmacology and Pathology, and graduated Alpha Omega Phi with an average over 90%. My USMLE scores were 99s and I recently matched in a residency for Family Medicine at Dartmouth Geisel School of Medicine. The improvement in my marks compared to prior professional school grades is remarkable.

The whole experience was a revelation for me. I thought constant daydreaming was normal. Up until this point, I would often phase out during times when I needed to pay attention or during things I thought were boring. I would just go home and learn the material on my own or miss important details. This worked reasonably well throughout grade school, university, and chiropractic college. But I never really enjoyed studying fully or doing things that I found boring. Studying was just boring. I also thought that work was boring for everyone, and that everyone hated their jobs for these reasons. I never understood how some people could focus in class and be so organized and create neat notes and schedules. I was never like that. I thought I would just remember important things and keep them in my head or just learn it later on my own. I now realize that I was working well below my potential all those years at school, work and in my life. However, I think I was able to get by in these areas because I was never really challenged enough to manifest my weaknesses as fully as they were during medical school.

David's Wellbutrin Experience

Wellbutrin enhanced meta cognitive functioning. The addition of Wellbutrin enhanced my ability to organize and prioritize information and tasks. For example, I could have several pieces of information either read or given verbally and I am able to recall them, prioritize and organize them now in a sequence that makes sense to me and then follow through on the task at hand. To that end, I am able to avoid hyper-focusing on a piece of information or idea/thought and move on to the next stage of problem solving with greater ease. An analogy would be adding an enhanced transmission to the engine (Vyvanse/Dexedrine) component. The Vyvanse/Dexedrine allows one to have the capability to initiate work (engine) and the Wellbutrin (enhanced transmission) then adds refinement to the work where tasks of greater importance can be prioritized and completed with enhanced efficiency.

In addition, Wellbutrin enhanced my verbal communication and listening skills. It allowed me to be more present during conversation, not interject at inappropriate times, and listen effectively to what the other person was saying to me and then react at the appropriate time with a natural response. I would liken this experience to listening to music with regular headphones and then listening to that same piece of music with noise cancelling headphones where the background ambient sounds are filtered out and the music is heard clearly and responded to as it was meant to be.

I also noticed that with the addition of Wellbutrin, my level of procrastination decreased. This is in relation to what I mentioned previously where I would sometimes become hyper-focused on a task or detail prior to starting Wellbutrin. The Wellbutrin seemed to remove this "mental stuttering" and created more fluidity of thought and task initiation.

David's Personal Statements on the Stages of Treatment

Upon initiating treatment with Dr. Hoffer, the dosage of Vyvanse was increased, which had a calming and balancing effect on my mood. I thought increasing the amount of amphetamine would make me feel too revved up thus making it more difficult to concentrate and focus. Interestingly, however, the exact opposite occurred. It is important to note that the amphetamine dosage was increased at the same time Wellbutrin was added to the treatment regime, so there was also probably a synergistic effect of this combination. Short-acting Dexedrine was added to take late in the afternoon which helped as Vyvanse had a tendency to wear off in late afternoon and it becomes difficult to sleep if more is taken later in the day. This combination has helped me feel the best I have in my life with regard to mood and accomplishing tasks that once caused much anxiety, worry and boredom due to the anticipation of procrastination and frustration whilst attempting to initiate and complete them.

Perhaps the most important component of treatment with Dr. Hoffer was the way he understands and explains to his patients that ADHD is a functional disorder. The analogy he uses is that of corrective eyeglasses. One can see without the lenses; however, they do not see as well as those with perfect vision. With much effort and strain, they can perhaps manage to get along not seeing 20/20, but eventually, they will miss important details and never enjoy the full rewards of having unimpeded vision. The individual can cope to an extent, but sooner or later their efforts will fall short, causing a vicious cycle of frustration, confusion, self blame, anxiety, depression, and eventually they just give up or give in.

This is in relation to the current theory of ADHD etiology. It is proposed that those with ADHD are deficient in levels of dopamine (DA) and norepinephrine (NE); the appropriate levels of DA and NE are the "corrective lenses" for the ADHD patient. When these levels of DA and NE are corrected to their normal levels in the individual with ADHD, they are then able to navigate their way through the world with less or perhaps without procrastination, dreading odious tasks, working more efficiently, and living a more productive life on all levels. The sense of dread and feeling overwhelmed they live with on a daily basis is alleviated and they can now live the life they were meant to live.

I feel that being educated properly about ADHD was just as important as having the correct treatment.

If I understand what is going on with my condition, then I better know how to manage it, what to expect, and why the recommended treatment regimen is required.

CHAPTER 14

Why is treating ADD so hard?

By now, you should have a decent feel for the strategic importance of addressing "both sides of the coin" in ADD treatment. In fact, this Stage I/Stage II approach is, for me, staggeringly obvious. Then why is it still not widely understood, accepted, and embraced?

There are a number of reasons, some of which I have already mentioned. But the lack of comprehensible treatment model is one major factor that inhibits and discourages physicians (including psychiatric and neurologic specialists) from trying to elevate the treatment outcome narrative. In other words, if you do not have a basis of understanding for what you are dealing with and how it can be approached in a systematic protocolized fashion, it always feels daunting, confusing, and overwhelming, which in turn makes it difficult to treat.

At the same time, it does not take more than five minutes of discussing ADD patients and their challenges and symptoms to have a roomful of doctors furiously nodding their heads in agreement that we absolutely must consider both attentional regulation *and* executive function regulation in patients. Anybody and everybody with any passing familiarity with ADD knows, both intuitively and pragmatically, that this two-pronged approach is a good idea, even if they hadn't articulated it to themselves.

So why is the Stage I/Stage II approach so radical? Separate from the glaring absence historically of a treatment model, the simple fact is that doctors don't know that the "other side of the coin" executive function (procrastination/motivation/decision-making) can be successfully addressed pharmacologically. Full stop. Why don't they know? All of the organization and time management and being aware of how you interact and how you are perceived and whether you can hit your pause button when you need to and make a better decision not to procrastinate when you really shouldn't and maintain, motivation and initiate — all of these function issues seem as if they are character traits. It runs against our central common sense to think otherwise. A person should just be able to will themselves to do better, get better, and be better. They should just stop being so effing lazy. Shouldn't they?

And therein lies the massive gulf in the ADD world. Everybody knows that this disorder comprises much more than a simple attention issue but almost nobody knows that the other accompanying issues can be dramatically and effectively addressed with medication treatment. There is a frightening downside to this ignorance. Because doctors are not addressing Attention Deficit

Disorder in this more complete and comprehensive way, the overwhelming majority of ADD patients *never* get the opportunity to achieve to a level commensurate with their ability and intellect. Never. Without proper treatment, the neurotransmission of their brain is never fully operative and engaged.

Is the problem as simple as what I have outlined here? Yes. It really is that straightforward. Does the combinational approach to treatment work for everybody? Absolutely not; nothing in medicine, and particularly in psychiatry, works for every patient. But this approach does work for the large majority of my patients. As well, there is more than just one treatment approach to consider if the straight line Stage I/Stage II doesn't yield a fuller and more robust treatment result. But to not consider trying this approach in a patient who has spent a life struggling with self-loathing and underachievement, unable to be effective in actualizing their hopes and aspirations, well, that is beyond understanding. It is time to get this story out into the world, to elevate the conversation, to get people, including doctors, to start offering a path for their ADD patients who never realized there was a way forward.

In the next few chapters, I outline cases that characterize examples of patient populations that require more than just the first two stages of treatment. I do so in order to enhance the understanding of the treatment model and how it can be applied to achieve even greater benefit to the individual patient. Not only are the cases interesting to read but they will build on your knowledge about the treatment of ADD. What is most important to remember, though, is this basic message: *Stage I, Dopamine, Regulation of Attention; Stage II, Norepinephrine, Regulation of Procrastination/Motivation.*

For the bulk of ADD patients who do improve with the combinational approach, the work is not done. There remains the need to continue with observation of benefit and side effect and tailoring of doses. When I sit with patients who have gone through the Stage I stimulant treatment and if required, Stage II norepinephrine enhancing treatment, and they are doing splendidly well, we review the five parameters that I want them to be aware of so that their treatment can be adjusted if needed.

These 5 parameters are:

1. focus / concentration
2. procrastination / motivation
3. mood / anxiety
4. getting along with others
5. being able to multi-task without getting flustered

The first parameter is generally stimulant-centered. If a person who is doing well starts to notice a diminution in their ability to focus and concentrate, that will generally require on adjustment to the stimulant dose and/or format or a switch from a Dexedrine-based medication to a Ritalin-based one (and vice-versa).

The second parameter relates to an adjustment of the norepinephrine-enhancing treatment (generally Wellbutrin in adults and Strattera in children). For those patients who are doing well on 300 mg of Wellbutrin every morning, approximately 25-30% of them will return to my office within a 3-month period and report that after a strong initial response of improved executive function, procrastination has reared its ugly head again. That occurrence requires an increase in the Wellbutrin dose to 450 mg (300 mg + 150 mg together in the morning). (Note that the top recommended dose of Wellbutrin is 300 mg in Canada but 450 mg in the United States.) Generally, if an adult patient does not have notable side effects on the 300 mg dose, they will likely not have significant side effects on 450 mg. If the increase to 450 mg works, I expect to see an improvement within 4-7 days. If no improvement occurs within 14 days, I usually return the Wellbutrin to 300 mg and deploy an additional augmenting strategy. (On rare occasions, particularly in patients weighing more than 150 lbs., there can be benefit in pressing the dose to 600 mg. The patient must be aware however that there exists a risk of lowering the seizure threshold).

In the ensuing three chapters, I will outline sequentially case examples that manifest assistance that can be provided to ADD patients who need "something more" to achieve a more complete result.

CHAPTER 15

Where does serotonin fit in and where doesn't it?

As I have detailed earlier, the majority of the adult patients I have diagnosed and treated, who were previously seen by one or more psychiatrists and/or psychologists and psychotherapists, were treated solely for depression. As shown, it is extraordinarily easy to slide these patients into the depression rubric. They almost all have low self esteem, are underachieved, are struggling with work and/or school and have significant problems in their personal relationships. They have what to be depressed about.

I cannot emphasize enough the importance of treating these patients, who present with comorbid ADD and depression, for their Attention Deficit Disorder first. In the majority of these cases, the depressive symptoms will dramatically diminish once the ADD treatment is fully optimized. What these patients need is to finally have the opportunity to function in their full state of capacity, which includes the ability to self-regulate, which in turns allows them to feel much more in control of mood, feelings, emotions, responses, and anxiety.

One always have to keep in mind, however, that psychiatric treatment, by its very nature, is not black and white. We use the term "comorbid" which implies that two diagnostic states can coexist in the same person at the same time. Just like you can have ADD and pneumonia, or ADD and a hangnail, a person can have both ADD and depression at the same time.

That said, the statistics that quote ADD comorbid with depression at 50-60% of patients is, in my opinion, both inaccurate and misleading. Inaccurate because I am certain that many of the people diagnosed with depression are suffering from low self esteem as a result of their inability to function properly in contrast to those (much fewer) patients who have a true coexisting depressive illness. Misleading because quoting those old (and broadly-accepted) statistics always leads doctors away from addressing the unfamiliar territory of ADD and towards addressing the more familiar issues associated with depression. Doing so usually results in an overall half-assed treatment result because the Attention Deficit Disorder remains untreated and ignored.

The most frequently used antidepressants over the course of the past 30 are SSRI's or Selective Serotonin Reuptake Inhibitors (such as Prozac and Celexa). What are they and how do they work? In the brain, our neurons (nerve cells) communicate with each other through chemical messengers called neurotransmitters. As a signal is transferred down the length of a neuron, that signal triggers the release of a neurotransmitter from its storage sac at the end of the neuron. The neurotransmitter is released into the microscopic space around the neuron it was just released from and floats over to attach to receptor sites at the start of the next neuron. The signal is thus propagated "down the line". Once the signal is sent, the neurotransmitter detaches from the receptor side to float back into the microscopic gap. [This gap is called the "synaptic cleft"; the whole connection is called a synapse]. The neurotransmitter is then vacuumed up or "reabsorbed" back into the neuron so it can be used again, hence the term "reuptake".

The result? SSRI's slow down ("inhibit") the reuptake (or reabsorption) of the neurotransmitter so more of it remains in the synaptic cleft. The releasing neuron senses that it is now somewhat depleted of its usual level of serotonin and sends a supply chain message back to the management center of the nerve cell telling it to start producing more neurotransmitter so it can maintain a steady state of supply.

Since the advent of SSRI's in the mid-1980's, they have been the most broadly used antidepressant group. They were, and are, an important addition to the psychiatric armamentarium. Not only were they a new option for treatment of depression, they also had a softer side-effect profile than the medications which preceded them. And, full disclosure, I used them a lot—as did nearly all of my colleagues. (I rarely use them now, for reasons that will become clear in this chapter).

SSRI's, like all medications, came with a well-established side-effect profile. The four "main" side effects are sexual dysfunction, fatigue, nausea, and weight gain. These are well known and most physicians will inform their patients, prior to initiating treatment, about them.

For adult patients on longer term (more than 4-6 months) SSRI treatment, there is another more subtle set of side effects that frequently occur. It is known as the "cognitive dulling" or "brain fog" that people will complain of. "Doc, I think I'm too young for Alzheimer's but lately I don't remember where I left my keys or parked my car. And I didn't get my taxes filed on time." Most doctors, pleased that their depressed/anxious patients are no longer complaining of depressive mood symptoms, usually reassure patients that this may well be a transient problem and certainly nothing to worry about. In fact, it can be quite problematic on its own but becomes more of an ongoing issue when it is accompanied, as it usually is, with a dulling or flattening of the patient's personality. "Doc, I'm not depressed anymore but in these past few weeks and months, I'm not able to enjoy myself like I should; I can't take pleasure or joy in my kids and in my family life, work has become a chore; there's no joy, no bounce to my step".

This is a serious problem. Anhedonia (lack of feeling) is experienced by people as a very troubling situation. They have no energy, they cannot sustain motivation, they procrastinate to their detriment, they can't initiate tasks or projects. Is this starting to sound familiar?

Wait, isn't this the chapter on serotonin? Yes it is. Neurotransmitters carry out their work in the brain among all the other neurotransmitters, hormones, and other chemical messengers, and they all subtly interact with each other. As well, the lack of energy and struggling with task initiation and motivation and procrastination problems all sounds very much like norepinephrine issues. Why would that be? The answer is simple but most doctors do not know about it: SSRI's down regulate and inhibit norepinephrine. As you've seen, everybody—and ADD people in particular—needs their norepinephrine neurotransmission to be working effectively to be able to fully function. Otherwise, one is always obtaining compromised treatment results leading to patients wondering, "What is wrong with me?"

Now let's consider the role of serotonin and mood/anxiety considerations in the treatment of Attention Deficit Disorder. If you ask me if serotonin has a direct role in ADD, my answer, consistent with my treatment model, is no, it doesn't. But do I frequently have to consider impacting the serotonin neurotransmitter to achieve a fuller and more comprehensive treatment outcome? Yes, I do.

The most frequent situation revolves around the patient who has been treated for both Stage I and Stage II treatment. The patient returns to my office for a follow-up appointment and reports that for the first time in her life, she is doing really well. Her attention is clear, sharp, and sustained. Her ability to be motivated and keep procrastination to a reasonable minimum is established. Time management, organization, and task completion are blessedly operating well for her. A common refrain is: "This is the best I've ever done; my functioning is great; I feel so proud and so much better."

But some of these patients, perhaps one in six, return and say instead, "Dr. Hoffer, if I knew when we started that I would end up functioning this well, I would have predicted I would feel terrific. But despite my significant improvement, I'm still not feeling all that great. I'm not exactly depressed or anxious, I'm just not feeling as good as I would have expected."

For those patients, assuming I have "tailored" their Stage I dopamine enhancing stimulant medication and their Stage II norepinephrine enhancing executive function medication well, I will then consider adding in a serotonin-enhancing mood improving medication. To avoid the potential down-regulating suppression of norepinephrine, I usually will not use the SSRI family of medications, though. Instead, I generally prefer using Cymbalta (Duloxetine) or Trintellix (Brintellix in the U.S., generic name vortioxetine).

Cymbalta is in the SSRI category, which stands for serotonin and norepinephrine reuptake inhibitors. Unlike SSRI antidepressants, however, Cymbalta enhances the availability of both serotonin and norepinephrine neurotransmitters. In so doing, it minimizes the tendency for serotonin to negatively impact the norepinephrine neurotransmitter, which the SSRI's (or "unopposed serotonin impactors" as I call them) do.

Trintellix (vortioxetine) is the other serotonin enhancing antidepressant that I also use frequently after Stage II for some patients. It is referred to as having a multimodal serotonin effect. While it does operate somewhat as a serotonin reuptake inhibitor, it mainly interacts with serotonin receptors directly. One of the receptors (a sub receptor) appears to have the capacity to block the serotonin tendency to down regulate norepinephrine, which results in the mood-improving and anxiety-reducing benefit of serotonin without the suppression of norepinephrine. Not surprisingly, separate from the world of ADD, Trintellix is tooled as an antidepressant that not only improves mood in a patient with depression but also can potentially provide benefits in cognitive capacity.

So when a person who I am treating for ADD needs to have some augmenting treatment in mood/anxiety, I will start on a low dose of a serotonin enhancing antidepressant medication (typically 5 mg of Trintellix or 30 mg of Cymbalta). Within 7-14 days, I have the patient report back to me. When this part of the treatment is successful, patients will report that they now feel "fine" or "better". Some will require an increase to the more standard dose of 10 mg of Trintellix or 60 mg of Cymbalta. It does not take more than 2-3 weeks to see improvement. (If the medication is well tolerated but not yielding any further clinical improvement, I will generally discontinue its use.)

The following patient, Dalia, is an example of a case which nicely reflects the consolidating benefit of having the last piece of the treatment puzzle added to the Stage I and II improvement.

"I am a 27-year-old female artist and in the past year I have been officially diagnosed with ADHD. This diagnosis has opened so many opportunities where I can finally begin to feel my true self.

I was born in former Yugoslavia and moved to Canada when I was five years old. I can remember when I was a child, constantly being bored but climbing everything in sight and still never really feeling satisfied. The transition to Canada wasn't difficult for me since I was young but it was blamed for my trouble in school along with a believed learning disability and dyslexia. I found school was a fun idea—all the books, pencils and textbooks, I enjoyed learning and never really felt unintelligent. I just couldn't sit there long enough to absorb the information given to me. Everything caught my attention and sometimes I felt like the lesson was going too slow and I just wanted it to be hands on or more entertaining and that seemed to be the best way to keep my attention. Having terrible memories of terrible teachers is really where I started to change my thoughts towards school and homework and I just began to dislike it.

I had my continued struggles but I continued with trying to push forward in life with little success and a lot of frustration with myself. It wasn't until my willingness to be open with a supportive friend where I explained my panic attacks, constant general anxiety, lack of motivation and lastly but mostly, my sadness and pain over all of this, led me to Dr. Hoffer.

When I came to see Dr. Hoffer, I proceeded to take a test and that's when he explained all my problems, pain and frustration, that I have had for what seems to be my entire life but which he saw just from that initial session, in just 5 minutes. I was honestly floored. I didn't know whether to laugh or cry, be excited or sad, but this was it. I was understood and I knew it was only going to go up from there on.

The next steps were all very informative on Dr. Hoffer's part. He explained how it all played out on the inside of my brain. He wanted me to know that information before we proceeded with the medication so that I could have a clear understanding of what he was trying to help me with and the medication he was going to prescribe. It was such a nice relief to know that a whole new journey was about to begin for me. Dr. Hoffer described how I would be able to focus, pay attention on what I wanted or needed to, finish my tasks, switch between tasks A through C and complete them with no issues. Once those started to improve, my mood and anxiety would also proceed to get better, and all of the issues that I've had would eventually feel as though they weren't a part of my life, that they were not who I was at all.

The first step we worked on was my focus and attention. I was prescribed Dexedrine because it also aims to help with my depression. Dexedrine unfortunately did not work well for me so we then moved onto the next medication, which was Ritalin. When I took it for the first time, I couldn't believe how I felt. I could do one or two tasks and not think about anything else but that. It was like my brain finally stopped with the overdrive, overthinking and overanalyzing about everything all at once. I felt at peace for the first time. I was simply able to finally sit down and write the content for my jewelry website in a matter of an hour, which was a surreal moment in itself. You have to understand that prior to that moment I had made numerous efforts to just begin the process of writing but to be able to sit down and actually write my first draft was outstanding. This was so different to me and unbelievable.

I'll be honest, my mood was still all over the place, which for me at times interfered with the focus and attention that I was finally starting to have. But I'm sure during the whole time I began the treatment, I was having a roller coaster of emotions from this new life change so I tried not to take every emotion seriously until I felt until things were stabilized.

Dr. Hoffer proceeded to prescribe Wellbutrin for my mood and ADHD, and slowly I started having less mood swings but it did take me some time to really notice because I was a bit of an emotional wreck if you couldn't sense that already. Finally, there was one last thing on the list which was that lingering sadness and lack of motivation, which had almost felt like a missing piece. That's when Dr. Hoffer prescribed Trintellix for my depression.

The Ritalin and Wellbutrin was for the dopamine aspect and finally the Trintellix was there for my serotonin aspect which was to bring it all together or as Dr. Hoffer would say, to finalize the last piece of the puzzle. Eventually, I began feeling happy and content, which at first was a confusing feeling, but then I began to realize this is probably how most people feel on a relatively consistent basis, and I finally had a sense of satisfaction and peace, which I had always struggled to find. Looking back, I feel lucky that Dr. Hoffer was willing to take me on and help me with everything. It has made a rather large positive impact on my life.

With the exception of a couple dose changes in between my treatment, which is common, I was onto my next journey.

In this past year of being diagnosed and treated, I started working full time, excelling into a leadership role and then landing a job in my field. My partner and I were able to buy a car and have a dog, and that is more than I have done in the past 6 years. I've gained a level of confidence that seemed to have disappeared along the way before; I am level headed and more in touch with myself than ever. My relationships with friends and family are flourishing and I can actually set goals and feel that I will get there—maybe not right at that moment but eventually.

With the help of Dr. Hoffer and his innovative perspective on ADHD and medication treatment, I have transformed from a scared and anxious individual who lacked confidence or self worth into a young woman where nothing can get in the way of my ever-expanding success."

CHAPTER 16

Where does Abilify fit in?

When a patient has responded well to the Stage I trial (and if needed, the Stage II trial), the change in their life is hugely significant. In a short period of a few weeks, the ADD person can do all the things that seemed so elusive to them. Where previously they would feel inept, disorganized, and unable to screen out distractions while trying to focus and concentrate, they can now smoothly and rationally sustain their attention, increase their productivity, initiate tasks and see them through to completion, and operate with more self-regulatory control throughout the day. The change can be profound and transformational. In fact, if I hadn't been doing this clinical work day in and day out for as long as I've been at it, I frankly wouldn't believe the possibilities.

As stated earlier, sometimes a patient returns to my office and reports that as good as the treatment responses has been—better focus, less procrastination, more motivation, being more tuned in socially—the patient feels "not quite there". They will go on, with urging, to describe some variation on the following theme:

"I'm certainly operating much better than I ever did before. Now when life comes at me one thing at a time sequentially, I can knock it out of the park. I never was able to handle things as well prior to getting my ADD treated.

But that's often not how life comes at me. Instead, things come at me three or four things at a time and then I become easily flustered and overwhelmed. I can't seem to be able, while already doing something, see something else come my way, target it, put it up on the shelf, finish what I was doing, and then take the next thing down from the shelf and apply myself to that."

I describe this "not quite there" feeling as "getting easily flustered while multi-tasking". Though not as concise a phrase as I'd like, it captures the functional "gap" that exists for a portion of the ADD population. Note that this is not a feeling that will be remedied by tailoring the dose of the first and second medications. Note also that this is not an uncommon phenomenon.

With increasing frequency, I find myself in discussion with patients about trying to fully augment the medication treatment of their ADD symptoms. But this challenge, being able to handle more than one issue at a time, is particularly important because it describes the regular challenges that people are faced with in their daily work/school/personal lives. Being able to operate smoothly and naturally in an efficient and composed manner is as accurate a description of an optimal therapeutic goal for a patient with ADD as I could formulate. As we think about "Attention Deficit Disorder", we are painting a more specific picture of the need for self-regulation.

Again, let's return to my office and I will outline what I say to my patients who require further treatment past Stage II.

The medication we can consider adding in to augment your treatment response is called Abilify, which is in a family of medications called atypical antipsychotics. At high doses, these medications are used for very serious illnesses—severe depression, schizophrenia, and manic-depression. At low doses, they are generally used to improve the response to an antidepressant medication.

Though Abilify is lumped in with the other atypical antipsychotics it is, in fact, in its own special category. The other atypicals operate by dopamine receptor blockade. They sit on top of the dopamine receptor and prevent the dopamine neurotransmitter from interacting with the dopamine receptor. These atypicals also are generally given in the evening before bed because of their two most common side effects, which are sedation and increased hunger. By giving them before bed, one hopes that the tiredness helps you sleep and doesn't persist into the working day. Similarly, we hope that you are hungry while sleeping and not overeating the following day.

Instead of being a dopamine blocker (or "antagonist"), Abilify is a partial "agonist" (meaning it sometimes blocks and other times facilitates the dopamine receptor). Abilify therefore acts to move neurotransmitter levels into the center zone, not too high and not too low. This "neurotransmitter modulation" quality is critically important to understand, as it appears to be both responsible for mood augmentation and enhancement of the ADD medication response that is already present. Essentially, the neurotransmitter modulation assists in "self-regulation" by moderating the levels of the operative neurotransmitters.

Abilify is given in the morning generally, as it usually does not cause sedation (tiredness) and is generally weight-neutral. Some people experience a bit of a mood and energy lift after taking it (good in the morning but could interfere with sleep if taken later in the day).

At higher doses of 15-40 mg of Abilify, there are other, more considerable side effects. But what we are talking about here are doses of approximately 2-4 mg. At low doses, the likelihood of significant side effects drops considerably. The side effects to watch for are dry mouth, feeling a bit "off" in the first couple of days taking the medication and occasionally fatigue. Though Abilify is generally weight-neutral, if combined with a serotonin enhancing antidepressant, the combination can slightly dull the satiety centre, that small part of your brain that lets you know when you are starting to feel full. As a result, eating just a little more at each meal can set up the patient up for weight gain. This potential side effect can be combatted by paying attention to portion control.

The final side effect is "akathisia" or motor restlessness. Rather than fidgeting with your hands, you notice this more as a legs issue, in which you feel compelled to always be walking around and you can't sit still at a desk or computer or dinner table. The chances of this side effect occurring at low doses, however, is remote.

I generally initiate treatment at 2 mg every morning for the first week. The patient then reports back to discuss the presence of any side effect issues and whether they have noticed any clinical improvement. For most of my patients, I will then have them maintain this dose for one more week and report back again. If they are somewhat better but feel they could do better still, I have them increase their dose to 4 mg (2 tablets) for the next week and have them report back at a follow-up appointment.

When this method of treatment works, the results are impressive. It often feels, to both patient and clinician, that the therapeutic outcome is complete. When I give talks to other physicians, I often outline the three items that my patients report at that point. First, they say, "I'm feeling better". They are experiencing a mood and anxiety improvement, which is mainly serotonin-mediated. That good feeling, I note, is not that surprising as Abilify has some intrinsic antidepressant/antianxiety activity and can support serotonin activity.

The second thing patients say after treatment is "I'm doing better". This comment refers to function/productivity/time management/ organization/motivation. The improvement here, I believe, results from the Abilify "modulating" the dopamine and norepinephrine neurotransmitters into a more effective zone.

Finally, patients report that "I'm feeling normal". I joke with people and ask, "How do you know what normal is like?" Their perfect reply: "I know it when I feel it."

These three outcomes—feeling better, doing better, feeling normal—represent the patient's more complete ability to function at a level more in keeping with their true capacity, intellect, and intentionality. For patients who have never had that feeling before, it is very meaningful. It allows them to start the process of being able to understand themselves as being fully capable, as complete and intact, instead of as the "damaged goods" feeling that has shadowed them all their lives. It allows them to very quickly get to know themselves in a more mature and composed way. It gives them a more smoothly operating "neurotransmission", which allows the various parts of the brain to start smoothly humming like a well-oiled machine.

The experience of a recent patient of mine demonstrates this result magnificently. A highly intelligent young grad student, underachieved to his intellect, was referred to me for a medication consultation for his quite significant "depression". In these next few pages, you will read his beautifully written summary of his experience. As you read it, take note of the following:

1. Keep in mind that the patient had previous experience with Wellbutrin, which yielded equivocal results as a stand alone treatment. Remember my explanation of how Wellbutrin works off the platform that the stimulant medication provides.

2. Observe how the sequencing of the treatment "builds" on itself. Sometimes I refer to this sequencing as "lasagna therapy" in that, in more complex presentations, I am layering one therapeutic agent at a time on top of the previous treatment.

3. Note the patient's own efforts, prior to diagnosis and treatment, to compensate and self-medicate, to try to "get by" and "get through". These are the "modus operandi" of so many young adults who have no idea why they can't do better than they are doing and why they end up feeling so helpless, overwhelmed, and "depressed".

4. Finally, watch how the patient emerges into what is manifestly a more "natural" state of being. I am the first to acknowledge how counter-intuitive it is to talk about a "natural" state when

multiple psychopharmacologic agents are being deployed concurrently. But then contrast his emerging "state of grace" with how he so clearly describes the state he found himself in previously.

"Throughout high school, I was able to succeed in spite of my study habits rather than because of them. I would consistently leave assignments to the last minute, needing the pressure of an imminent deadline to inspire the dedicated concentration required to complete them. Studying for tests followed a similar pattern, as I relied on my ability to successfully cram the information I needed, usually only a day or two before a test. These inefficient habits were not openly problematic in high school, but it quickly became apparent that they would not lead to success in undergrad. After a very mediocre performance in my first year, I slowly improved my work ethic enough to find much more success in the following years of undergrad. However, I still found myself frustrated with my tendency to procrastinate and poor ability to plan, which very often made assignments and exams much more difficult than they needed to be. Through it all, though, I graduated in four years with high honours, and after an unsuccessful bid for medical school, decided to enter a Master's degree program.

In the first months of my degree, the concentration and work ethic issues that were manageable in undergrad quickly became much more detrimental. Without the schedule of regular assignments and deadlines and the seemingly endless amount of time ahead of me, I began to spiral into a pattern of extreme unproductiveness. I would spend hours at my lab each day, mindlessly browsing the internet at my desk, and half-heartedly doing impressively little actual work. Time began to pass, and by the end of my first semester, I had become aware that a serious problem was developing. My supervisor's concern grew as I consistently had very little to show for myself with each passing month. The essays that I was able to complete in a day or two in undergrad had become comprehensive reports that required weeks of effort. Effort that I was not able to give on a consistent basis. I began to miss deadlines and fall further and further behind.

As months passed, the situation began to take a serious toll on my mental health. The sight of my supervisor caused me anxiety and panic. Thoughts of my future turned from optimism and excitement to dread and frustration. My attitude toward the degree became that of hatred and anger. I wished I had never chosen to do it. I felt trapped in it. And despite all this, I still could not find anything in myself to change, which eroded my belief in myself, my abilities, and my self worth. As week after week passed without significant accomplishment, I sank further and further into depression.

I had first encountered marijuana in undergrad. Every so often, my roommate and I in first year would walk to a nearby park to share a joint, then return to our room to watch funny YouTube videos. Throughout undergrad, it was merely something I would partake in when the opportunity arose, such as the occasional party. I never bought it for myself, and thus it had very little effect on my studies. After a year of my masters though, a friend of mine introduced me to a nearby dealer. Suddenly, weed took on new life as an escape from the hellish circumstances of my degree work. When I was high, my crushing pessimism turned to optimism. Life felt good, and I believed in myself. Quite simply, it made me happy, which was not a familiar feeling anymore while sober. Of course, despite these feelings, I still had no will to work when high. All it really did was remove the shame of it. As the habit became daily, things became even more dire. I was going weeks getting absolutely nothing done, and being constantly high made this behaviour feel perfectly acceptable. When I tried to quit, the crushing weight of reality and the shame of my failure to perform would drive me back to it. Somehow, I had become very addicted to a drug that I once considered totally innocuous.

Through all these circumstances, I reapplied to medical school and was interviewed by a nearby university. At first, I was placed on the waitlist, but in early June of 2015, when I was supposed to be finishing my degree, I received a call saying that I had been accepted to the school. I quickly transitioned from ecstatic to panicked as I realized that my acceptance was conditional on the completion of my masters by August of that summer.

In a meeting with my committee a few days later, I broke down crying as everyone in the room collectively realized that I had very little to show for myself after two years of work, and the notion of completing the degree in two months was impossibly optimistic. Nevertheless, my supervisor and I helped draft a plan to collect the necessary results and create a defendable thesis by the deadline. In the initial subsequent weeks, I was determined and focused, believing that I could accomplish the goal and realize my dream of becoming a doctor. But when July came, my mood began to plummet at the prospect of the impending deadline, and in my despair, my productivity fell once more. I again turned to marijuana and the self-sabotage that only compounded the problem and effectively ensured my failure.

Though the school offered me an extension of two weeks, I had completely broken down by early August. One day, without consulting anyone close to me, I completely lost my composure and told the school and my supervisor that I was quitting the masters. In my mind, the degree was causing me immense emotional pain, and I couldn't bear the thought of being in it any longer. Obviously, I lost my offer and was left in total despair, made worse by the fact that my family and friends strongly advised me to continue to try to complete the degree, as not doing so *would only further deteriorate my prospects for the future.*

After a short break, I returned to my degree work that fall, but my mental health was extremely compromised. I frequently ideated about suicide and felt a constant self-loathing. Even worse, I returned to my marijuana habit with even greater dependency, purchasing a vaporizer, a device that creates a vapor of the drug that can be inhaled much more easily than smoke, and creates nearly no residual scent. I began to use the device constantly, in my office and at home, as it made it extremely easy to hide my use from my supervisor and from my girlfriend at the time.

A couple months passed of this constant use, all the while accomplishing quite literally nothing of value, until on a day of unusual sobriety I had what can only be described as a complete mental breakdown. Locking the door to my office, I made a noose from an Ethernet cable and hung it from the coat rack on the back of the door. As I let myself experience the sensation of the cable softly pressing into my windpipe, I realized that I was in serious need of help. I called my brother in tears and confessed my despair. He in turn called my mother, who insisted that I come back home to Denver to get healthy again.

In Denver, separated from my lab and the surroundings that I associated with my internal hell, I recovered a bit. I started seeing a psychologist again, and slowly began writing again, a little bit each day. The process was painful and difficult, but I began to build a bit of momentum and to start rebuilding things. Unfortunately, by this point the already strained relationship with my girlfriend had reached its breaking point, and when I returned to Toronto two months later for the new year, we ended our nearly six-year relationship. Despite this blow, I still made a concerted effort to improve myself and finish my degree. I began seeing a psychologist regularly to stay on top of my mental health, and though I could not purge marijuana from my life, I was able to find a semblance of control over my habit.

However, I was still struggling immensely to be productive, and still felt quite depressed. After a few months, it became clear to my psychologist that I needed medication. He referred me to a psychiatrist he knew, Dr. Mayer Hoffer. Initially, I was skeptical about seeing Dr. Hoffer. I had seen multiple psychiatrists in the past and was never overly impressed. I had tried Prozac, which had done nothing during the time that I went through my medical school failure and subsequent breakdown, and Wellbutrin, which improved my mood initially but did not seem to change anything significant. Dr. Hoffer, though, asked me to write about my experience and explain why I was seeing him, which intrigued me. I had never known a psychiatrist to go so in depth into my life and struggle. Upon reading my story, he gave me a very surprising conclusion: I suffered from ADHD. Initially skeptical of this diagnosis, the more he described how it related to my issues, the more sense it made. I had always had issues with procrastination and focus, and particularly over the past two years, my ability to concentrate on my degree work was extremely compromised. He told me that my issues with concentration and productivity had led to my depression, which resonated with me. I became convinced when I took my first dose of the medication he prescribed, Dexedrine. Quite suddenly, I was able to engage and focus on my work. I was able to run and keep track of multiple experiments and spend much longer amounts of time working in the lab. I felt like a productive human being for the first time in ages, and my mood improved.

However, after a few weeks, I began to falter again. When I did work, I was effective, but I struggled to get myself to work in the first place. My mood began to fall again, and I felt the negativity returning. At this point, Dr. Hoffer prescribed Wellbutrin, which seemed to improve things slightly, but not significantly. As spring turned into summer, I became increasingly despondent about work again. My goal at the beginning of the year had been to finish by June, but June came and went and I still did not feel close to the finish line. As I faced the prospect of failing yet again, my mood began to plummet severely. I was on medication that was supposed to help me succeed, and yet I was still not the person I wanted to be. I thought myself broken, useless, and hopeless, and with that, suicidal urges returned with frightening intensity.

At this extreme low, I saw Dr. Hoffer once more. He offered me few options for a next step, recommending a low dose of Abilify to add to my drug regimen. I was obviously pessimistic about how effective this would be as well as slightly reluctant to be on medication specifically labeled as an anti-psychotic. However, I took out the prescription and began taking the drug.

I must emphasize that I am not being hyperbolic when I describe the changes that took place. Within only a couple of days of adding Abilify, the change I experienced was nothing short of miraculous. Suddenly, I felt like I was looking at the world with a clear and balanced head. The things that were causing me intense feelings of despair and hopelessness were now simply stressful challenges that I felt confident and motivated to meet. I woke up in the morning on time and began having full and productive work days. I not only felt happy, I felt normal. I felt like I could handle the world and take on challenges and approach life the way I wanted to. For the first time in years, I was not depressed. My productivity soared, and as I write this, I am finishing up the final stages of my thesis draft, with the goal of defending in the coming weeks. And unlike previous times, I am self-assured in my ability to meet this goal. I feel like the effective and successful person that I was in undergrad, and I feel excited for my future. Wellbutrin and

Abilify have stabilized my mood and helped make me confident and motivated, while Dexedrine has helped me realize my working potential and accomplish my goals. I am extremely grateful for the help Dr. Hoffer has given me, and I hope my story is able to help others in my position."

CHAPTER 17

What role does Intuniv play?

When I come home at the end of the day, I empty my change into a plastic bag. Other people keep it in a piggy bank or a coin jar. When my bag gets heavy enough, I lug it to the local grocery store where they have an automated coin counter. I've tried to imagine how the machine sorts the various coins. In Canada, we have toonies and loonies (two dollar and one dollar coins) as well as quarters, dimes, nickels, and pennies. I imagine that inside these machines there are a series of five or six trays that automatically sort the coins by size.

Similarly, my ADD treatment model can be seen as a series of filtering trays or stages. Some of my patients only require the "Stage I" treatment that enhances their dopamine-mediated attentional regulatory issues. Give some assistance to the dopamine neurotransmission and those first stage patients are "good to go". Others, who need help with their norepinephrine-mediated procrastination-motivation issues fall through the first filter onto the second tray. Provide those people with help enhancing their norepinephrine neurotransmission and you are off to the races. In the preceding two chapters, I have gone past those trays and explained the third tray (serotonin) and the fourth (neurotransmitter modulation).

In this chapter, we turn to the role of Intuniv. Just as each of the "trays" brought forward something separate (but interconnected) to consider, the fifth tray does as well. Of course, we don't have to use all of these treatments at the same time. There is a "mix and match" process that leads to a tailoring to suit the individual patient but that requires an understanding of each tray (or level) and what it potentially offers.

Intuniv (Intuniv XR) is a medication that I deploy across the life cycle. Though it is only specifically approved for children and teenagers, I prescribe it to adults of all ages if their clinical presentation "coins" filter down to this fifth "level" (or tray).

As explained earlier, Intuniv is built like an anti-high blood pressure medication (the medical term is antihypertensive). Its mode of action in the ADD area is not dependent on its effect on blood pressure. Rather, it facilitates the smooth transmission of signals through the frontal lobes of the brain. The frontal lobes, which are the seat of self-regulatory control and management, are then able to function in a more efficient and effective manner. Intuniv doesn't immediately start to show clinical results; it takes approximately 10-14 days to start to manifest clinical improvement. Intuniv can be used as a stand-alone treatment but it is most often used in conjunction with a psychostimulant.

When it works, I patients tend to report one or more of the following five observations:

1. My thinking is sharper and it is qualitatively different than just an increase in focus and concentration

2. I am more composed. I feel more in control of my decision-making.

3. I am more productive. I am getting more accomplished.

4. I feel that I am getting my act together. I am more organized and effective in what I am doing.

5. I get along better with the people around me at work and at school. I am smoother in my interactions.

Intuniv does not have many side effects. The only of note, which are both mild and generally ameliorate within the first week or two, are fatigue and feeling somewhat lightheaded when standing up quickly.

Generally, I start with a 1 mg tablet in the after-dinner period (you could start it in the morning as long as the fatigue side effect is not pronounced). If the medication is well tolerated, after one week (in adults), I increase the dose to 2 mg. At the end of the second week, the patient reports on progress. If the direction of the treatment is positive, we continue on 2 mg for another week before increasing to a 3 mg tablet. Most of my adult patients are on 2 or 3 mg; a few are increased to 4 mg.

What is notable about the dosing regimen for adults is that it is identical to the dosing requirements of teenagers and children. I believe this is because the medication acts as a facilitator for neurotransmission. Once the signals are transmitting effectively, more facilitation doesn't help the signals become any more functionally efficient.

Since some patients' overall executive function is not helped by Wellbutrin and/or Abilify or there is sensitivity to side effects, Intuniv is a good third option. It provides ADD patients with another path to achieve a fully and more comprehensive treatment outcome. In my estimation, it is a very important option (albeit a second or third choice) if a patient is still struggling with procrastination/motivation issues even if the stimulant medication has a positive influence on attention.

That said, where I find myself deploying Intuniv more and more is after I have already initiated treatment on both sides of the ADD coin. I will have my patient on the Stage I stimulant treatment to enhance focus and the preferred Stage II treatment (Wellbutrin and/or Abilify) for a period of a few weeks or months. They then come back and report to me in a follow-up appointment; remember at that point that these patients have already experienced significant improvement in their day-to-day functionality. If they report that they are maintaining an excellent level of function, the treatment doesn't change.

However, if they say, "I wish I could be a little sharper" or, more particularly, if they say "My attention and motivation are really quite good but I could still improve in how I am getting along with others," Intuniv may be the next best option. In well over half of these patients, after 2-3 weeks of an Intuniv trial, they will return to my office and report a further step up in their overall clinical improvement. This beneficial effect is due to the enhanced "neurotransmission" impact that the Intuniv is providing.

A perfect clinical case example is that of Kevin, an adult man who came to my office many years ago. He had always viewed himself as a nice but distinctly inferior person. As a child, he had been identified as having "LD" aka learning disabilities. He had always been in the "slow class" at school. Not a great student, he managed to get through and obtained steady employment after dropping out of college.

On formal psychological testing, some 50-60% of ADD people will be diagnosed with a learning disability. You would think that this puts ADD people in a further disadvantaged position. In fact, many doctors, upon hearing that a patient has both ADD and LD, feel that it is too daunting and complex a case to handle.

In fact, it isn't. If a person with Attention Deficit Disorder has a coexisting learning disability, the most crucially important clinical imperative is to treat the ADD. Why is that?

Let's take an example from my life. I am not the most gifted handyman. When I come home at the end of the day, if Mrs. Hoffer says to me, "This broke today; please fix it," well, let's just say that fixing things is not my area of strength. So what do I do? I try to figure it out; I call up my friend who actually has tools; I drop by the local hardware store; I read up on the problem. In other words, faced with a relative area of weakness, I whistle and call upon my areas of strength to help me compensate and cope.

A person with an LD is a person with an area of relative weakness. We all have these areas and we try to compensate as well as we can for them. But the difference is that a person with ADD and LD, when faced with an area of weakness, whistles to call upon areas of strength that don't come running. It's as if they are "not paying attention".

There is a reason that I am oversimplifying the very complex field of coexisting Attention Deficit Disorder and Learning Disabilities. I do so because in some 90% of cases, if you treat the ADD, the person with ADD and LD improves dramatically in their functionality and ability, including marks in school and productivity at work.

Have I "cured" the LD by treating the ADD? Absolutely not. Have I enabled the patient to whistle and call over their areas of strength to buttress their areas of weakness so they can operate like most capable and effective people? Absolutely.

What happens to people like Kevin with diagnosed Learning Disabilities (and undiagnosed ADD) is that they grow up from early childhood with a palpable concrete sense of being not good enough and not smart enough—in everything they do. School, work, friendship, self-esteem. Everything.

When I met Kevin, he presented with the usual mix of low self-esteem, dysphoria (mild depression), inattention, disorganization and frustration. The overwhelming likelihood is that a young man in his late 20's exhibiting these characteristics will be diagnosed with depression and prescribed a serotonin-related antidepressant. Now we are back to the depression/anxiety "tray" that I referenced earlier.

Kevin clearly had "both sides of the ADD coin" in his presentation. He was inattentive and easily distracted. He could not sustain concentration for longer periods of time. He was a chronic procrastinator and was unable to maintain motivation when required. I explained to Kevin that we needed to address his Attention Deficit Disorder first and then see what else might be needed after that.

And so, over a period of some years, Kevin's ADD was successfully treated, starting with Stage I, and he responded with improved attention. Stage II treatment then addressed his procrastination/motivation issues, and his executive function significantly improved. Some years later, to boost the overall response, we added low dose Abilify to his treatment protocol and he improved further, being more able to multitask without getting flustered.

He was so much better than he ever was before. Finally, he was able to see himself as the intelligent, capable, and compassionate human being he had never been acquainted with. He was vastly more successful. Sometimes I illustrate this post-treatment experience as patients finally shaking their own hand and getting to know themselves for the first time in their lives.

And yet, Kevin felt he wasn't all the way there. He still had difficulty with smoothly sensing the social oscillations around him. He was using his brain better than ever but not all of his cylinders were firing smoothly. So to this treatment regimen, we added Intuniv

XR at 1 mg to start, then moved after a week to 2 mg.

Kevin, who was already significantly improved prior to the Intuniv, started to report that he was experiencing a more complete and comprehensive improvement. He was more tuned into social nuance and interaction. Instead of being socially awkward and hesitant, he became more confident in his interpersonal interactions and benefitted by making new friendships. He felt more "in system" with his academic work and clearly became more productive. He felt that we had found the final piece of his "ADD puzzle"—the piece that allowed him to operate more successfully socially and academically.

A final note. Kevin is not only a high achieving Master's degree university graduate now, but he is also a leading social community activist, advocating for the poor and dispossessed in our society. Fancy that.

CHAPTER 18

Where is my confidence?

My patient population is dramatically diverse. I see young children and senior citizens, foreign students from Asia and suburban soccer moms, real estate agents and teachers, business executives and unemployed people on disability. Attention Deficit Disorder cuts a wide swath through every layer of society but no matter who you are, if you have ADD, and you decide to proceed with treatment, I have every expectation that you will improve. In fact, I explicitly tell all my patients that they should expect a big improvement. Why would they take medication, and why would I prescribe it, if they were only going to experience a minimal and modest change in their ability and capacity?

Once a person in my practice starts to improve, two somewhat contrary experiences often occur. The first is mixed emotion, a combination of surprise that something actually seems to be working, hope for the future, delight in being able to concentrate, and sometimes anger that they were never given the opportunity to have their functional challenges understood and treated previously.

The second emotion is fear surrounding the erosion of confidence. This fear is illustrated by the typical question that ADD people ask me once they see improvement. They wonder if it will take as many years as it took to treat their Attention Deficit Disorder to now recover their confidence. The rest of this chapter will address the impact that the chronic erosion of the foundational underpinnings of confidence has on ADD people of all ages. And how that can completely change for the better.

For children with ADD, the central questions start early. "Why am I so different than everybody else? Why can't I get things done easily and regularly and in the expected time frame? Why can't I make friends easily? Why can't I keep friends? Why aren't I invited to birthday parties? What is wrong with me?" For more inattentive and less impulsive children, the so-called "daydream inattentive" presentation, the sense of being ostracized and marginalized socially, may be somewhat less but the questions remain the same. *There is something wrong with me.*

These questions beg for answers. Teachers tell the ADD child that he needs to try harder. Parents call him lazy. Other people tell him he is dumb or crazy. Other parents tell their children not to play with the bad kid causing trouble at school. Siblings avoid him, calling him annoying or just hit him. The child feels angry at being criticized and shunned and then wonders if he is crazy and bad for being angry and this is why others don't like him.

In adulthood, ADD people have become very familiar with

their limitations. Many have just chalked it up to "that's who I am; take it or leave it". Others have worked furiously, often to the point of exhaustion and strain, to try to compensate for their weaknesses. They draw up schedules, they put reminders into their smartphones, they colour-code their to-do list. But the gnawing central experience remains. I am not as good as other people. I am not as good at getting things done. I am not as smart as others. I am not as smart as I used to think I was. I wasn't in the line-up when the royal jelly was being handed out. I am just not as good.

The natural consequence of this process is a staggering undermining of confidence and self esteem. It is almost always accompanied by a gnawing sensation that although the ADD person can sometimes put on a good "show" of being personable and confident and in control of a situation, it might all fall apart in an instant. The bottom line feeling that ADD people experience is that they are plagued by self-doubt and uncertainty and have to expend huge amounts of energy trying to cover that up. It is why, when the "surface" starts to "crack" and things fall apart, the ADD person can become quickly very flustered and anxious or angry and irritable and blaming others for their failings. It is also why they so often, almost automatically, receive the diagnosis of "depression and anxiety".

Many of my ADD adult patients have shared their feeling that the "show" they put on at their jobs is a veil that they fear their manager/boss/co-worker will look behind only to discover that there is nothing there. They view themselves as an empty shell with no substance behind their "song and dance" routines.

Needless to say, this kind of day-to-day experience is a lousy way to live one's life. Moreover, it is inaccurate. People spend their entire lives thinking, "This is who I am and there's nothing I can do about it." And the saddest part is it's not a true representation of who they are—and they don't even know it.

After completing the initial assessment, I tell a new patient that he is very likely not the inferior incapable morass of poor protoplasm he has always feared he is and that he will soon have the opportunity to get to know a much more capable and successful 2.0 version of himself. I know that upon hearing this prediction, the patient believes I am displaying either naïve optimism or the height of presumptuous arrogance. After all, how could I predict that outcome if I've only known him for an hour or two? But I have seen the same case over and over. Each patient will finally get the chance to really get to know him or herself—the able, capable, competent, true version of self.

When people start to improve, I review the process and timeline that will unfold with respect to the repair and restoration of their confidence and self-concept. This discussion represents a separate non-medication role that psychiatrists, psychologists, psychotherapists and ADD coaches can also play in this process. No matter the patient's age, they will go through what I call the "3 levels of confidence", which takes 4-5 months in total.

The first level happens during the first month of treatment. At this point, something clearly good is going on, maybe even great. The patient starts to feel that a significant change has occurred, particularly with respect to their ability to focus and concentrate. They are hopeful and excited but the dramatic improvement reminds them of other times in their life when they thought that they were on the right track but then everything fell apart after a short while. Appropriately, they remind themselves to reserve judgment and remain sceptical and somewhat guarded. At the first level of self confidence building, something good has happened but the patient can't help but feel that maybe this is just a trick that will fade.

The next confidence level is achieved in the following two months of work and/or school. Of course, for patients who are unemployed or off work on disability or not in school, the time frame is slower as they are not getting the chance, on a daily basis, to meet and succeed at work challenges. In this second and third month of treatment, people start to see that they can do very good work, they can be organized and productive, and they can avoid procrastination and sustain motivation through to task completion. They get the opportunity to see that not only are they able to operate in a capable, efficient manner but they can do just as well as the "regular effective people" that they always use to wish they could be like. By the end of the second level, they also see that they can rely, day in and day out, on their treatment working, that it's not a trick that fades.

Now obviously the second level sounds pretty good. Most people (including me) would want to sign on the dotted line for that level of improvement in function and confidence. But there is a third level that's even better. In the fourth (even fifth) month of work and/or school, the patient starts to experience stronger confidence in their executive function. At this stage, the expression I use is that "it doesn't matter what they throw down on the table in front of you that day, you can eat right through it."

The other "tool" that I deploy in the process of helping my patients in the restoration of their confidence is pointing out the success that they experience. I know that sounds odd; after all, success is the goal that you aim for. But for ADD patients, getting the chance to experience regular reliable "leave it with me, I'll get it done" success actually becomes one of the tools that can help them try harder, dig deeper, climb higher because they never had it in their hands before. Once they get the chance to operate to their capacity, they can do great things. And they can get to know who they really are.

To give you a more clinical feel for this process of restoring a person's confidence as their Attention Deficit Disorder is recognized, diagnosed, and treated, meet a 31-year-old real estate agent, who was referred to my office for a diagnostic assessment. In her history, she noted that she had been diagnosed with a learning disability as a child. Suffering from focus and memory problems leading to anxiety and stress, she was at her wit's end but was obviously both personable and articulate. At the time of the initial assessment, she was not on any medication.

This patient had struggled in school but had graduated, with effort, from high school. She entered college with enthusiasm but dropped out soon after. She suffered with bulimia during her teenage years but that had finally resolved as she entered her twenties. She had been treated with the antidepressant Prozac for depression at age 16. She had also seen a therapist two years previously for "depression". Her family psychiatric history revealed alcoholism on both sides as well as a brother with Attention Deficit Disorder.

Her mental status examination revealed a self-conscious young woman who described her mood as "generally anxious". She attributed this anxiety to the stress she experienced when she would feel unprepared for tasks and then would become quickly flustered. She was clearly more intelligent than her school history indicated. She imagined that her friends would describe her as a "good friend but flaky". She subscribed to almost all of the 18 ADD diagnostic criteria as noted in her Adult Self-Report Scale.

After dropping out of school, and after a few short-lived jobs, she decided to make use of her people skills and become a real estate agent. She was able to get through her examinations by working very hard. As the course material got harder, she "borrowed" some of her brother's psychostimulant medication, proudly noting that she got 97% on her final licensing examination.

In the first session, she noted feeling very overwhelmed. "I can't remember what I go into a room for or where things are. I struggle to pay attention to details. I have to go over things numerous times and I still don't get it right. All of this makes me anxious".

She noted that she had struggled with alcohol until two

years ago, but had been able to moderate her drinking to 3-4 glasses of wine per week. She "fought" her weight and believed that if her life was more in her control, she would be able to better integrate regular exercise into her weekly routine.

When I inquired about her procrastination/motivation issues, she replied that her tendency to avoid and delay completing tasks that she knew she needed to attend to was at "an all-time high even for the simplest task." Now that she was working as a full-time commissions-only real estate agent, her procrastination was an insurmountable impediment and a source of huge stress for her. "My life is a real mess."

Before outlining how her treatment unfolded, permit me to emphasize three points. Had this woman seen any number of my psychiatric colleagues, she would have been treated for "depression and anxiety." After all, she was not a "jumping bean", she was pleasant and conversational, and she was female and distressed. She was anxious and lacking self esteem. Depression and anxiety. Anxiety and depression.

The second point is that she had a long list of clues pointing to Attention Deficit Disorder. She struggled to pay attention. She was hugely disorganized and unable to prioritize. She fulfilled DSM-5 criteria for her ADD symptoms. She had a first degree relative (her brother and likely her father) with ADD. And, although this is more a "Hofferian" criterion, she had demonstrated the "first year college collapse syndrome" that I always ask about. Frankly, a case like this not being diagnosed with

ADD by a psychiatrist or psychologist drives me just about crazy because it is so obvious and it is so important for the patient to get properly diagnosed and treated.

The third point may be the most important of all, although it is potentially confusing. More than anxiety and depression, and even more than attentional issues, the patient's history chronicled a difficulty being able to self-regulate. Here was a young woman who had a hard time regulating her food intake during her teen years. Difficulty regulating her attention. A struggle with regulating her decision-making and prioritization. Trouble feeling like she could self-regulate her mood state. A struggle to self-soothe and regulate anxiety. Difficulty managing self esteem and confidence. Difficulty regulating time management. I think you get my point.

Now perhaps if there were a diagnosis of Self-Regulation Dysfunction Disorder, there would be a broader, clearer understanding of the clinical picture—and perhaps more acceptance by both the medical profession and the general public. Here, "SRDD" would be more pertinent a diagnosis than anxiety/depression and even ADD.

Following her ADD education session, the patient decided to commence medication treatment. Starting at a low dose and tailoring upwards, she was on short-acting Dexedrine tablets, reaching 1 ½ tablets in the morning and after lunch and 1 tablet in the later afternoon. Her side effects were negligible. The benefits were large and obvious:

- "I'm definitely a lot more productive."

- "My thinking is clearer."
- "My "hyperness" has gone down; I'm able to remain very composed."
- "I'm able to get started better in the morning."
- "Procrastination has not been as much of an issue."

This was a strong start and characteristic of the proper direction of the initiation of Stage I treatment. Her dose was further tailored upwards to 2, 2, 1 ½ (2 tablets after breakfast, 2 tablets after lunch, 1 ½ tablets in the later afternoon). Seen 9 days later, she reported negligible side effects and a further significant enhancement in clinical benefit ("improved therapeutic ratio"). She was "a lot more focused" and noted being less fidgety. She felt her motivation was improved but her lifelong tendency to procrastinate was slightly better though still prominent. I instructed her to maintain her current dosing regimen and to report back in a few weeks. Doing so would allow her to clearly observe executive function deficits and, at the same time, consolidate her sense of her new "baseline" day-to-day functionality.

Three weeks later, she reported further improvement. Procrastination issues had lessened further. She was feeling really good — "work is amazing; so productive; more confident; I feel better about myself." She was also benefitting from the initial success she was experiencing. I often talk about early clinical gains being almost like an additional therapeutic device in the patient's "tool-belt" which elevates the person's unfolding development.

The other noticeable improvement was in the way she presented herself. She was manifestly more confident and was able to address topics more directly. Without sounding too new age, her aura was different; she had evolved more. She was starting to operate more like her true self.

Despite the improvement, I sensed that she was likely to head to Stage II treatment down the road. But there was no need to rush as she was so clearly improved, and waiting, while observing her for a few weeks, was the proper and prudent course of action. I don't just give people the Stage II treatment because I have a protocol; I give Stage II treatment to address a "neurotransmission deficit" if there is one.

Two weeks later, the patient reported that her procrastination issues were "still kind of there" and interfering with other aspects of her improvement. Again, the point of ADD treatment is not to just get the patient somewhat better; it is to give her the opportunity to operate naturally at the level she is biologically capable of. This patient was already better. In fact, she was a lot better. But still, she was capable of so much more.

What has routinely happened to ADD patients in the past, if they were fortunate enough to get treated at all, was that they would emerge only partly better after treatment. Then, after a period of time—a few weeks, perhaps a year—the frustration at never being able to really "get going" would lead them to abandon medication. They quit not because it hadn't worked but because it wasn't nearly as helpful as it needed it to be. It is this frustration that leads many ADD sufferers to experiment with drugs and alcohol because they are seeking different answers to the same problem.

The patient was started on Wellbutrin XL 150 mg every morning for 1 week. After that time, she called to report that she had no side effects of note and had already started to see improvements in her executive function. She was stepped up to 300 mg for the next 8 days and then arrived at my office for the next appointment.

Her result was both characteristic and outstanding. "I have more clarity and focus. I just do instead of sitting and dwelling on things. I am much more confident. My procrastination tendency is almost gone. I am more motivated." She noted no side effects. She felt very proud of herself. She looked transformed—more composed, more self-assured, and beaming.

There was no mistaking it. She was already well into the second level of confidence.

CHAPTER 19

What happens if it stops working?

When I was training to be a psychiatrist, ignorance prevailed in the field of Attention Deficit Disorder. Of course, I didn't know that at the time; I had to find that out for myself many years later. There were some enormous misconceptions about ADD—it is a boy's problem only, everyone outgrows it, it doesn't exist, it's not important anyway. When you are young and in the education system, you are taught that it is proper and respectful to accept what your teachers tell you, even in medical school.

One of most dangerous points of misinformation was the thinking that it doesn't t matter whether or not you treat ADD because these patients all end up doing badly anyway. Leaving aside the colossal therapeutic pessimism that such a position represents, this "clinical fact" has given the psychiatric profession a free pass for far too long. After all, why work to treat a condition that doesn't respond to treatment efforts anyway? And, by the way, who knows if it even exists? In other words, why even bother trying?

Now, as you have read here so far, my practice runs counter to this perspective in every way. My unshakeable clinical position is that I fully expect to achieve a huge improvement in my Attention Deficit Disorder patients in both the long and short term. There are tremendous transformational changes that occur when a person finally gets a chance to focus and pay attention and get started and achieve goals and have a life and become proud and confident. I've seen it time and time again.

But as I've noted, not every patient gets better. Almost all of my ADD patients will improve but a large number of them will need to have their treatment adjusted along the way, in the same way that cars need a tune-up now and then. That's just the nature of the practice of medicine.

Then there is the patient who has a good therapeutic response and, after some time has passed, returns to say the treatment is just not working nearly as well as it was, or even not at working at all. This drop in response is so disheartening to an ADD patient who finally, after a lifetime of failure and doubt and underachievement, experiences a good or even great response to treatment. Now, after months or years of success, that patient returns to my office with a doleful expression and tells me he fears he has regressed to the way he used to be.

In this situation, we are seeing an example of "tolerance", meaning your brain has become less responsive to the therapeutic effect of the medication so the dose is no longer effective. Tolerance is common, according to the literature, and can occur in approximately 30% of cases.

So here is a hell of a situation. According to the "experts", it doesn't really matter if you get treated or not because the outcome is going to be dismal anyway and oh, by the way, if you are being helped, you have a 30% likelihood that the benefit will fade and disappear.

Allow me to set the record straight. True "tolerance" is much more of a rare occurrence and certainly nowhere near the quoted percentage. In my experience, what is too often referred to as "tolerance" is simply the failure to "tailor" the dosage of stimulant medication appropriately. Over the years, I've had many patients, who were treated with a starting dose of stimulant (18 mg of Concerta or 20 mg of Vyvanse, for instance), come in for a consultation because the referring physician states that the patient has become "tolerant". What I see is not tolerance. Rather, it is a simple failure to have adjusted the dose over time to a more appropriate one.

Then there are those patients who claim their stimulant treatment is no longer effective, reflected in the resumption of their original symptoms of inattention and distractibility. What do I do with these patients?

All of the medications I have been writing about are ultimately expressed through neurotransmitters, the chemical messengers in the brain. Neurotransmitters connect with neurotransmitter receptors. These receptors are quite specific and respond to their particular neurotransmitter "partner" in the same way as a lock responds to a certain key. It is thought that tolerance occurs over time perhaps due to "receptor fatigue". In other words, the receptor gets tired and stops working.

For real tolerance, there are four strategies. The first is to try a slightly higher dose, which sometimes works right away. Another option is to switch formats. Instead of a long-acting stimulant, sometimes patients will react better to the short-acting stimulant given once every 4 hours (or vice-versa). The third option is to stop the stimulant for a few weeks and then retry with the hope that the receptors will have "refreshed" themselves. Finally, the fourth and often the most effective strategy is to switch from one stimulant class to the other stimulant class (change Ritalin to Dexedrine or Concerta to Vyvanse and vice versa). Making this switch allows for uninterrupted treatment and is often useful for a period of time. In fact, some of my patients need to "cycle" every few months between the two stimulant classes.

When we consider patients for whom the medication seems to have stopped working, they are often people who have a more complex ADD presentation and are on three or more medications. Almost always, these patients also have a clear past history of depression and anxiety prior to their ADD treatment. What do I do in these cases?

For years, I would do what I always do—adjust doses, change formats or delivery systems, switch antidepressants, and whatever else I could think of. I also tried referring to other treatment modalities, including counseling, coaching, and exercise, for instance, but in these patients, doing so did not help.

Every so often, a patient presents with a clinical challenge that forces you to think harder and reach deeper. Such a case presented to me recently, and it compelled me to shift my conceptual thinking. This was the case of a young woman in her first year of university. She had been my patient since her mid-teens. She had been treated for serious depression by a respected psychiatrist in the community with little success. She and her parents were referred to me on a "last hope" basis.

She was a lovely young lady in great distress and torment. She was very intelligent but had missed chunks of the school year due to periods of feeling sad and overwhelmed. She also had significant ADD issues, which she had compensated for with her intellect. I adjusted her antidepressant medication regimen while I initiated her ADD treatment following my Stage I/Stage II protocol. Fortunately, she started to improve, and steadily, over the next few weeks, she was able to resume attending school, seeing friends, and generally having the positive and functional life she was meant to have. Over the next three years, with no specific periodicity, she would have a few weeks when her mood would become dysphoric but, with adjustments to her combination of medications, she would resume her now successful life as a teenager attending high school.

When she went off to university, it felt like a huge milestone had been reached. She was proud and excited and I was very happy for her. Shortly after, however, she returned for a visit and reported that the medication had seemed to stop working. I reviewed her treatment then outlined how we could adjust a couple of her medications higher to try to achieve a better outcome. With each adjustment, there was a brief few days of improvement followed by the same phenomenon—the medication seemed to stop working. Understandably, the patient was scared she might return to the very dark place of her mid-teens and I was both fearful for her and confused by this alarming and sudden loss of treatment effectiveness.

Over the course of a few days, I racked my brains trying to understand what had happened. Was there something I had missed? Was there an adverse drug-drug interaction that I was unaware of, where one medication creates a toxic and negative effect in the patient when another medication is present at the same time? And why, given that she was on a combination of medication for both ADD and depression, had everything stopped working at once?

For reasons that I can't articulate, it struck me that the most heuristic and straightforward explanation for this conundrum was that the medication had simply stopped being delivered to the sites of action in the brain. Or, more properly stated, the blood flow to those parts of the brain that the medication needed was not sufficient enough to deliver the therapeutic quantity. There is evidence that the perfusion (or blood flow) of certain parts of the brain is relatively reduced in psychiatric illness states. This reduction can be demonstrated by certain types of brain scans. Think of it this way. If the neurotransmitters are akin to the "transmission fluid" of the engine, then not having an even distribution of blood flow would be akin to deficiency of oil in the engine. When a psychiatric illness state is successfully treated, the "democratic perfusion" of the brain is restored.

I consulted with a marvelous colleague of mine, Dr. Mary McLean, who agreed with my perfusion deficiency concept. We both felt that the likeliest medication, which might restore more equally distributed blood flow, was an anti-seizure medication called Gabapentin (trade name Neurontin). Though it is used in the treatment of epilepsy in quite high doses, for our purposes, a lower dose would likely be sufficient. Since this medication is also occasionally used as a "mood stabilizer", psychiatrists are familiar with it. I settled on a treatment regimen:

- Day 1-5 – 100 mg every morning
- Day 6-10 – 100 mg every morning and evening
- Day 11-17 – 200 mg every morning and 100 mg every evening

I told my patient to report back every few days. I also told her that this was not likely to work but seemed worth a try since the side effects were minimal and there was some association with Gabapentin evening out cerebral blood flow.

Within two weeks, my young patient was back to her previous full functioning. She was in a good and steady mood, was able to pay attention, and demonstrated her full decision-making capacity. There was no "eureka" moment, but rather, a gradual and steady return to function, which she steadily maintained for the rest of the school year.

This was a remarkable result and hugely lucky to boot. I also cannot emphasize enough that a single anecdotal result, a "one-off", really means very little in clinical psychiatry and medicine. But what happens in the clinician's thinking very soon becomes something like this: Even if that treatment was lucky, I wonder if it might be helpful in other similar cases or in those cases that aren't doing nearly as well as I would have expected.

The fact is, it is through the process of exactly what I just described that improvements to the field occur. In the clinically based world, you observe a problem, you wrestle with it, you try to figure it out, maybe then you try something. If it works once or twice, you may have something. If it works frequently and you've tried it 30-50 times, then you have a new angle of thinking and attack. The caveat is that at all times, clinicians must remain fully mindful of never trying a course of action that would jeopardize the health of patients.

There was a difference, though, in my "discovery" of the utility of Neurontin. Unlike other times over the years when I observed improvements and then worked backwards to figure out why it produced a benefit, this time I was starting with a new proposition—that of adequate perfusion. I felt intuitively that this is the physiologic basis for why these patients improve but I had no "laboratory data" for my supposition. Still, I strongly believed in this new angle of attack.

As a result, I started using Gabapentin in other patients who had struggled to maintain their therapeutic improvement. Over the course of approximately 18-24 months, I have had significant improvement in approximately half of the patients that I have treated with this medication. While this result may appear to be less dramatic than other treatment protocols I have outlined, it is not. Given the fact that this is a "tougher" group of patients (patients who had previously not responded as well), this yield of improved treatment response is much higher than anticipated.

From a clinical perspective, the treatment protocols that I have outlined are as solid to me as concrete. My treatment model is that firmly constructed. As you've read, there are many factors that have led to my confident presentation—the great success of my patients, the many decades that I have been working on finding treatment for ADD sufferers, the fact that my treatment decisions, which are based on the treatment model, yield obvious improvements consistent with what the model would predict. Some may still view me as a delusional kook or consider my understanding to be only partly right due to the limitations of the current state of science and medicine. Still, protocols I have created must be shared so that the discussion of the very widespread condition of Attention Deficit Disorder in the field of medicine can finally move on from 1970's thinking.

This final "sorting tray" treatment, the addition of a medication to enhance and equalize blood flow throughout the brain, has a very attractive aspect to the conceptual treatment model. Although I am using it as the final step in ADD treatment in difficult cases, it could be argued that perhaps it should have a higher ranking in the order in which a medication is introduced. Because I have only been deploying Gabapentin for the past two years, instead of decades like most of the other treatments, the simple answer is I don't know. At least not yet. My clinical intuitive sense, my gut feeling, is that this medication is not required earlier in the process simply because if the other treatments are working, by my definition, that would imply that the perfusion of the brain is adequate enough in the majority of cases. But this idea of equalizing blood flow earlier in the process is certainly one to consider going forward.

CHAPTER 20

What happens in real live cases?

When my children were little, I spent many enjoyable bedtimes reading books with them. One of their favourites was the *Encyclopedia Brown* series, which outlined the exploits of a 10-year-old genius boy detective. Each chapter detailed a challenging case, which Encyclopedia would have solved by the end. If you couldn't figure out how and why he found the answer, there was a page at the end of the book that revealed the critical clue that determined the solving of the case. In these next two chapters, with thanks to Encyclopedia Brown, I present a series of cases that will clarify the thinking process, based on the treatment model, that helps to guide my clinical decisions.

CASE #1 CHALLENGE: The Case of the Underachieving Procrastinator

Nicholas was a 34-year-old machinist from the Indian subcontinent. He was treated in his late teens by an ADD specialist with psychostimulant medication. He noticed a significant improvement in his attention on a combination of two Dexedrine 15 mg spansules in the morning (which have a duration of action of 7-8 hours) followed by two 5 mg tablets of Dexedrine after school to help with studying and homework. Still, he was plagued by severe procrastination issues, which meant he never fully achieved his goals and aspirations. The previous specialist tried to deal with his motivational deficiencies by pressing ever higher with his Dexedrine doses but his procrastination challenge remained. Moreover, as his stimulant dose was increased, he became somewhat irritable and noted unpleasant side effects of appetite suppression and sleep disturbance.

After a few years, his doctor moved away and his treatment lapsed. Despite his ambition to attend university, he could not muster enough initiative to stick with school, eventually finding work as a machine tool apprentice.

When he came to see me, Nicholas had not been treated for a dozen years. He was very intelligent and articulate but felt his impulsive verbal style had interfered with his ability to maintain social relationships. He also noted lifelong difficulties with organization. He said, "These issues have plagued me for many years. I am at the stage in my life where I would like to move forward from these things. I want to reach my full potential."

Because of his former positive response, Dexedrine tablets were prescribed, starting at a low dose and moving up to 2 tablets at breakfast, lunch, and in the later afternoon. On his return appointment, he noted significant improvement in his concentration but little change in procrastination. There were no side effects of note. What would you do now? And why?

CASE #1 ANSWER:

By this page of the book, the answer should be obvious. Nicholas had a long prior history of response to stimulants to help improve his attention. But he had never had more than a "half-a-loaf" response. Nicholas clearly needed a Stage II treatment trial in conjunction with his Stage I treatment so as to impact "both sides of the ADD coin".

CASE #1: So what happened?

Nicholas was prescribed Wellbutrin to help assist his norepinephrine mediated procrastination/motivation issues. Within three weeks, he was vastly improved—more organized, more attentive, reporting more successful social interactions and improved memory. His procrastination was significantly reduced and much more manageable. He had no side effects and felt he was getting his life back on track. Over the next 9 months, he was maintained on his medication regimen (Dexedrine 5 mg tablets – 2 tablets three times a day and Wellbutrin XL 300 mg every morning). He reported advances at work and better personal relationships and described his treatment response as "transformative".

CASE #2 CHALLENGE: The Case of the Lazy American

Steven was referred to me by his family physician. A year earlier, he had moved from Boston to Toronto. A 44-year-old photographer, he been struggling to gain traction in his professional career for many years. The family doctor's consultation request was very informative:

Please see 44-year-old male for assessment and management of ADD, depression and anxiety. Recently moved from the United States. Saw psychiatrist while there and medication regimen as follows:

- *Concerta 36 mg caps – two caps every morning*
- *(Ritalin) Methylphenidate – 15 mg every afternoon and 10 mg every evening*
- *Ativan 0.5 mg tablets – 2 tablets as needed for sleep*
  Patient tapered off Concerta and Ritalin several months ago due to increasing anxiety and irritability but finds his concentration is very poor and affecting his daily activities.

Tried one selective serotonin reuptake inhibitor antidepressant (Zoloft) in past. Stopped caring about things; felt very flat so did not continue. Given concurrent conditions and side effects of medications, psychiatry consult and follow-up greatly appreciated.

In the material Steven prepared for his initial visit, he wrote the following:

Past Experience: Past Diagnosis, What Worked, What Didn't

- *Diagnosed with Attention Deficit Disorder as a teenager. My parents didn't tell me until I was an adult. They didn't medicate me.*
- *Struggled with school, didn't go to college.*

- *Re-diagnosed 2012, and was prescribed Ritalin, Concerta and Lorazepam. I had monthly appointments with ADD specialist in Boston, which really helped. He helped me understand the benefits of the medication and helped me overcome my reluctance. We discussed strategies for working with ADD that worked for me, such as having consistent routines, putting things in the same place, doing things at the same time, eating the same healthy foods, exercise, sleep, having healthy patterns for myself.*
- *I noticed immediately when taking Ritalin that it was much easier for me to read and track conversations. Less impulsivity. Anxiety at times. Used Lorazepam as needed for anxiety and for sleep.*
- *Things that were difficult: Although I was healthy, I noticed that the medication raised my heart rate. When I first moved to Canada and got married, the stress and the medication led to overwhelm. Concerta would start to wear off at 8 hours.*
- *I use meditation and mindfulness, which helps with impulsivity.*

Goals: What Do You Want to Change?

- *To have a consistent, workable treatment plan that includes medication and finding new strategies.*

In the consultation meeting, Steven presented as a thoughtful and articulate fellow. He told me he had finished high school but quickly found college too difficult and dropped out. He went into the army shortly after that and spent the next three years there. He had a series of jobs helping to run businesses but had not stayed for very long at any one job.

He reported a clear history of difficulty sustaining concentration and reading, and problems tracking conversations. He had huge problems with "IMP" issues (impulsivity, motivation, and procrastination). His mood was relatively "okay but with some anxiety". He was frustrated with his lack of achievement and feared he was "just lazy". Recently married, he wanted to get his life on track.

The rest of his history was unremarkable. His physical health was good and he had no significant history of drug or alcohol abuse.

Steven's case is classic. He was smarter than how he had ended up doing. He had the classic collapse in his early experience at college but had done better in the structured army environment. He had gotten "one side of the coin" treatment in Boston which, though it showed some benefit, did not touch the impediments he experienced on the Stage II issues of procrastination, motivation, and initiative. His frustration ultimately expressed itself as "anxiety" and the smart and well-intended family doctor then placed him on an unopposed serotonin impactor, which not only did not help his anxiety or mood but also classically "flattened" him by "down-regulating" his norepinephrine neurotransmitter—the very substance that would need to be enhanced and facilitated in order for him to improve.

CASE #2 ANSWER:
STEP 1: What did I do first?

Though I frequently start patients on short-acting Stage I

stimulants when I am initiating treatment, Steven had a clear previous history of the "paradoxical response" to a stimulant. He also, more recently, had experienced some adverse side effects to his Ritalin and Concerta. Because of this, I started him on a trial of Vyvanse (once daily Dexedrine), starting at 20 mg and increasing every few days upwards to 80 mg, which is the equivalent of the 72 mg (2 36 mg capsules) of the Concerta he used to take.

Steven had an excellent initial response to his Vyvanse medication. He described the following benefits:

- *"I didn't fight with my wife all weekend."*
- *"I was more pleasant to be around."*
- *"I noticed the house was dirty <u>and</u> I cleaned up."*

As his dose approached 80 mg, he noted:

"The biggest benefit is my improved capacity to relate to my wife. I now have just enough buffer time to think about what I say to her, which makes a big difference."

Steven also noted that though he was "able to see tasks through more easily,", he still struggled with motivation. Fortunately, and not unexpectedly, he had few side effects from the medication.

STEP 2: What did I do next?

Having followed along with the "Hofferian" protocol, you can likely guess what I did next. I initiated the Stage II effort, building on the Stage I platform, by prescribing Wellbutrin XL to enhance the norepinephrine neurotransmission. I started Steven on Wellbutrin XL 150 mg every morning (in addition to his Vyvanse 80 mg) and after 10 days, increased his dose to 300 mg.

Seen three weeks later, he noted further significant improvement in his executive function. He was able to prioritize better, his tendency towards procrastination was further diminished, and he felt he was on the right track. His mood was good and he felt more motivated. He was taking on more projects. He still felt that there was even more that he could accomplish but he was doing very well. I encouraged him to wait and observe himself, and report on his wife's observations as well, while he consolidated his gains and monitored his new baseline.

One month later, while still achieving better than ever before, we agreed to increase his Wellbutrin dose to 450 mg every morning (consistent with U.S. dosing guidelines but above the Canadian guideline of 300 mg). Seen two weeks later, he noted two minor side effects. He was sweating a bit more than usual (which later dissipated) and he occasionally felt a bit "flooded" (which indicated that he was still adjusting to being more productive).

The benefit was strong. Steven was starting tasks and seeing them through to completion. "I don't leave things undone anymore," he noted. He was keeping lists and noted he was more socially engaged.

One month later, in follow-up, Steven reported that he was significantly further improved and much more engaged, with no adverse side effects. The only remaining issue he identified was that he could still get "stuck" in the course of his day. He could still be better at prioritizing when a lot of activity was coming at him.

THINK ABOUT IT: What would you do now?

This case underlines just how crucial it is to understand the underlying process that likely accounts for the clinical picture that presents. One could argue that at this point in his treatment, a doctor should not offer anything more to Steven other than to maintain and monitor his successful treatment because to do more would be too aggressive and even reckless. Why put the patient in any jeopardy by adding anything else when the treatment is working?

There is certainly merit to that approach. But before you get too comfortable, keep in mind that the same rationale could have been used at any point along the way to justify a much less impressive and satisfactory-to-the-patient response. After all, Steven was feeling "better" on just the Vyvanse alone. In fact, he was already "better" on half the dose of Vyvanse as well.

The issue is not whether Steven, or any other ADD patient for that matter, can "get better". The question is whether, by using skill and understanding, and observing a living breathing treatment model, you can enable the patient to achieve to the true level of their natural ability. I had already helped this patient a lot but his treatment is not about me as the doctor. It is solely about this patient and whether he is now fully enabled to live the life that he is manifestly capable of living.

I started Steven on a trial of low-dose Abilify as follows: 2 mg for the first 2 weeks, followed by an increase to 4 mg as there was initial improvement with no side effects of note. The rationale centered on these facts:

- He required slightly more enhancement of his executive function.
- He was already on a significant dose of Wellbutrin.
- He had had a negative response to a serotonin antidepressant agent.
- Abilify could very likely facilitate the "fine tuning" of his response through its neurotransmitter modulation quality.

CASE #2: So what happened?

Steven had a superb response to this treatment regimen. He not only felt fully capable, but he also noted that the Abilify seemed to smooth out the therapeutic ratio (benefit vs. side effect) throughout the day. Moreover, he noted being steadier. "I feel kind of normal now," he mused. Seen over the next year, he maintained his outstanding response. The only change made to his medication was a reduction from 4 mg to 2 mg of Abilify after about 6 months.

Problem solved.

CHAPTER 21

How do we treat complex ADD?

Now that we've examined some of the more classic ADD cases, let's turn to two that represent what I call "Complex ADD". By complex, I am referring to the fact that the fine tuning of the treatment result required more adjusting over the course of time. Because the clinical picture can shift as some challenges are dealt with and others emerge or become more prominent, the treatment process takes longer. In both of these cases, the treatment ended up including anti-anxiety and antidepressant medication, but my job was to fine tune the relative levels (or proportions) of the neurotransmitter milieu.

CASE #1 – Andrea

Most adult patients only realize that they have ADD when their child is diagnosed and treated. Andrea was 46 years old when she decided to speak with me about her own struggles, some 8-9 months after her young son had become my patient. She was already familiar with my treatment approach and had seen significant improvement in her child's behaviour and functional capacity.

Andrea presented as someone who had it "all together". She was perfectly coiffed and attired in a manner befitting her top level management position at a bank. In her own words, she described herself as follows:

"As a child I was very hyper and unable to focus and participate in organized school class room activities. I was in trouble a great deal, made poor grades and had few friends who could tolerate my impulsive, hyper behaviour.

In my late 20s, I was doing poorly working in a structured corporate environment and realized that if I did not learn to better organize my work and myself and stop being so hyper, I would continue to perform very poorly. I became over-structured and organized, took project management courses, practiced acting calm and attentive in meetings and took copious, detailed notes to help me remember things.

My hyperactivity subsided as I got older but I still use the same tactics of being very structured with project plans, task lists, check lists, detailed notes and listening tactics. Despite these efforts, my work is very disorganized and I often lose important documents and forget critical deadlines or procrastinate until it's too late to complete work with good quality.

I am a senior leader at a bank and as my work and responsibilities become more complex, I am struggling to follow and organize my thoughts on execution and my impulsive decision-making often causes poor choices, incomplete and effective solutions and is limiting my career. My managers have pointed to lack of focus, impulsive and poor decisions in actions as a performance issue. My inability to follow complex concepts and issues greatly hinders me and has held me back from work opportunities. At home, I have very little patience with my family and have a great deal of stress in chaotic, unstructured situations. I have strong emotional outbursts in situations of conflict, which occur daily in my family life. I find I have very poor self esteem and am sensitive to criticism and tend to overstate my knowledge or act like I know something I have only limited understanding of.

I want to be able to focus, listen and think more completely before I make decisions, react or say things. I want to be able to follow complex concepts and feel more capable in my work and my family life. I want to reduce my stress in dealing with conflict or in disorganized or chaotic situations and stop biting my nails."

The rest of the history was, for the most part, standard issue. Andrea was physically healthy and had no particularly striking aspects of psychiatric illness in her family of origin. She had never previously sought out counselling assistance, choosing instead to rely on her smarts and her determination. Her difficulty sustaining attention and coping with procrastination issues had been present since childhood. She "hated school" and had dropped out of university fairly quickly. Fortunately, she found work at a large financial institution and had thrived within the structured environment. She was happily married to a supportive spouse and was living a busy and at times stressful modern urban life, that included a job, marriage and children.

From the outside, this was not a terrible picture. In point of fact, this woman had done much better than most adult ADD patients would have. She didn't have a drinking problem, she wasn't on her third marriage and fifth job, she was financially solvent. But her feeling of always being on the verge of it all falling apart was palpable. As her life became more complicated, her ability to compensate by treading water ever more furiously was resulting in her feeling overwhelmed and exhausted. She described how her feelings of low self esteem and inadequacy had worsened with her mood becoming more challenged. In my consult note, I wrote "obvious adult ADD" and noted that she would need Stage I and Stage II treatment.

Andrea initiated treatment with Dexedrine 5 mg tables and was tailored upwards to 1 ½ tablets after breakfast, 1 ½ tablets after lunch, and 1 tablet in the later afternoon over an 8-day period. She had some minor side effects in the first week, including a slightly dry mouth, reduced appetite, some minor impatience, and occasionally a feeling of being "caught in the moment".

The benefits were striking. "I feel like I am able to tap into my brain like I have never been able to." She felt more "in the flow of things" at work and at home. Her mood was lifted. She was more productive, even though she wasn't exactly jumping on things.

Seen two weeks later for her next appointment, she had settled at the lower dose of 1 tablet three times a day, as the 1 ½ tablet dose left her feeling in a slight daze. "I feel good but I am noticing being a bit disengaged; I am not as willing to get into things." Her early motivation had lessened and she was experiencing more of the old tendency to procrastinate.

As per my protocol, Wellbutrin XL 150 mg was initiated and, after two weeks, it was increased to 300 mg every morning (in addition, to 1 tablet of Dexedrine 3 times per day). At first, Andrea noted a great improvement in her organization and productivity. However, this was followed by a feeling of having a hard time tracking people's conversations in meetings at work. I wrote in my clinical notes that things for her were improved but "not quite right".

Remember that the medications that are being utilized are impacting brain function; they are psycho-active. Even if they are beneficial and on target, the central nervous system has to get comfortable and more familiar with what this feels like. Most patients describe the feeling as relatively natural, partly because it often results in early and encouraging dramatic improvement.

I decided to lower the dose to 150 mg alternating with 300 mg for a week. She was more comfortable one week later and then we decided to press back to 300 mg for the following week. Now her problems following conversations had gone away. The benefits were larger, too—her energy level was higher, she was always thinking ahead, her motivation was stronger, she didn't procrastinate, she was very busy at work, and she got along better with her co-workers. "I feel brilliant at times," she noted, which was quite a statement for a modest person.

Andrea had an outstanding treatment response. We jointly decided to maintain her treatment for the next month and a half to provide some time to consolidate the gains and establish her new baseline. In her follow-up appointment, she reported the same benefits, but noted a tendency toward a quick temper. She requested a switch from her three times a day Dexedrine dosing to the once daily Vyvanse. (Remember that Vyvanse is essentially the same

Dexedrine molecule in a slow release format).

Andrea started on a 20 mg capsule of Vyvanse (the equivalent of half a tablet of Dexedrine given three times a day) and after a few days, increased to 30 mg every morning (at ¾ of a tab three times a day equivalent, slightly less than 1 tablet three times a day of the tablet form she had previously been on). She felt more patient and calm but "a little dopey" when seen two weeks later. It was decided to tailor her stimulant dose up to 40 mg.

She was well maintained for the next few weeks. However, when seen one month later, she noted she had "had a rough week" in the week leading up to her appointment. "When I feel good, I feel really good but I frequently feel low and lack confidence," she said, pointing to the trigger as an "emotional conversation" she had engaged in with her boss. Because of her tendency to experience some dysphoria and anxiety, we decided to add a low dose of the antidepressant/anti-anxiety medication Cymbalta to bolster the serotonin neurotransmitter that assists mood and anxiety symptoms.

Andrea reported improvement in her overall mood and, seen a month later in early June, she felt a general improvement in the stability and reliability of her overall state (both ADD and mood aspects). Her medication regimen remained the same for the next couple of months except for an increase by August to 60 mg of Cymbalta to help bolster her overall mood and state.

By the end of August, her mood was good as was her focus. She handled day-to-day stress in a more efficient and confident manner. She felt she was doing well at work but noted occasionally having a hard time organizing and getting started on work projects. What, if anything, should I have done at this point in the treatment?

Andrea was in a much better state with her treatment than she had ever been before. She had an excellent therapeutic ratio: great benefit versus negligible side effects. There is an excellent case to be made that nothing more needed to be added to or changed in her treatment regimen. In fact, leaving everything as is was one of the considerations when she and I discussed her treatment options.

The overriding factor was that Andrea wasn't operating to the level of her potential. The struggle with task initiation in particular was not commensurate with her strong improvement in her executive function. This challenge, coupled with her history of dysphoric mood, led me to augment her treatment with low dose Abilify (2 mg).

Over the next three months, Andrea flourished. Her mood was better, her ability to start/continue/complete improved, and she experienced a very productive period at work. Now this was a very successful outcome. But even terrific treatment results require monitoring and modification over time. We had already adjusted Andrea's treatment but there was one more change coming.

At her next follow-up appointment, Andrea told me that her overall capacity was still strong. But there were two problems she noted. The first was a 7-pound weight gain. The second was a general sense of feeling flat and not taking pleasure in the course of day-to-day activities.

Now these two problems may be seen as being a consequence of the addition of the Abilify (in conjunction with a serotonin-enhancing antidepressant like Cymbalta, there can be dulling of the sensitivity of the satiety center, which alerts a person when they are full, thereby resulting in weight gain). However, what was more likely to be the "culprit" in her side effect situation was the tendency of serotonin-related antidepressants to down regulate or suppress the norepinephrine neurotransmitter activity. Such an impact results in the flattened anhedonic (pleasure lacking) experience that patients experience after a few months of taking an antidepressant.

That does not mean that Cymbalta is a bad medication. It means that both doctors and patients need to understand the importance of the interaction of their medications to help guide their treatment and the consequences that result. In Andrea's situation, the temptation to see her "flat feeling" as "part of her depression" would in many psychiatric offices result in an increase in her antidepressant dose, which would result in exactly the opposite of what was intended, as doing so would have left her feeling more flattened and led to further weight gain.

What did I do? I put Andrea on a "cross-over" plan in which I tapered down her Cymbalta dose and then discontinued it while ramping up her dose of Trintellix. Trintellix is a unique antidepressant that supports serotonin (through a different mode of action than Cymbalta) but does not result in a suppression of norepinephrine. It also appears to avoid the weight gain that can occur in conjunction with Abilify.

What happened to Andrea? Pretty much precisely what you

would expect. She became happier and felt much less flattened. Her energy was better; she felt more engaged. There was no increase in weight or appetite. "I am much more clear-minded, particularly in the afternoon," she noted.

Her case serves to emphasize, yet again, the importance of having a treatment model and understanding the interactions between the neurotransmitters. The model always guides treatment decisions above yielding vastly improved clinical results.

CASE #2 – Jonathan

Jonathan was 24 years old when he came to see me four years ago for a consultation assessment. He had a good job with an international management consulting firm. He had been assessed the year before by a psychologist and was told he had "obsessive thinking, which is an adult form of Attention Deficit Disorder". He had been started on 40 mg of Strattera, which was only partially helpful.

Jonathan was plagued by "living too much in my head." He noted he had too many thoughts and spent too much time trying to sort them out. As a result, he felt he was "not alert, not in the present". He was not a good listener and felt that he was not as creative and productive as he could be. He had significant problems maintaining his focus if he was not interested in the subject matter. He always left things to "the night before" but would "figure out a way to get things done." He found himself always having to read things over again a few times to fully grasp what was on the page. He noted his brain often felt "foggy".

The only other part of his history that was notable was he had a number of mild concussions while playing football and hockey, which resulted in a post-concussion syndrome with daily headaches for one year. He had been seen by a neurologist and had an MRI of his brain done, which was normal. He had no history of seizures. With support and tutoring, he had been able to graduate with his Bachelor's degree at university.

This patient's prior treatment with Strattera is something that I commonly see when a patient is diagnosed with ADD but the treating physician does not want to prescribe stimulant medication. Almost always, this decision is based on a lack of familiarity with stimulants, coupled with the desire to avoid using a class of medications that many doctors feel is controversial. As discussed earlier, Strattera is both "approved" for ADD treatment and is a "non-stimulant", which many doctors find attractive. Unfortunately, on its own, Strattera generally is not as effective a treatment as the Stage I/Stage II treatment approach. In comparison with stimulants, Strattera improves dopamine neurotransmission only weakly and it is not as strong a norepinephrine enhancer as Wellbutrin is. Hence, patients on Strattera alone frequently note that their response to treatment is only a partial one.

Within two and a half months of our first meeting, Jonathan was clearly having the classic Stage I/Stage II response. He had no side effects and noted "my head feels very clear." He was much more productive at work and felt he was functioning very well. He started to make plans to return to school part-time to get his executive Masters in Business Administration (MBA). A few months later, he was settled into a routine of using Vyvanse 50 mg every morning, Monday through Friday for work, and Vyvanse 40 mg on weekends (along with his daily Wellbutrin). Doses higher than 50 mg left him feeling uncomfortable.

A few months later, Jonathan felt he had "plateaued" somewhat and could use some extra assistance with procrastination. A trial of increasing his Wellbutrin dose to 450 mg yielded little benefit and he was returned to the 300 mg level.

Approximately one year after our first meeting, we decided to try to boost his overall effectiveness by adding in a trial of Intuniv XR. What was the rationale? Jonathan was already doing better in terms of his daily ability and function. But he was astutely aware that he was not yet achieving to his full capacity—likely because his ADD treatment was not fully effective and also, there may have been a lingering residual symptom of his concussion history.

My thinking about Jonathan's case is as follows. His dopamine/attention issues were addressed as were his norepinephrine/procrastination issues. By adding in Intuniv XR, which has minimal risk of side effects (he was clearly sensitive to small changes in dose), we could have the smoother neurotransmission that may repair and reset the "slower" foggy signal transmission. I may very well have added in Intuniv XR even without the history of head injury; the point is that there was a clear rationale for considering it.

What happened to Jonathan? With the addition of Intuniv XR (eventually settling on 3 mg), Jonathan reported being more attentive with a clear reduction in "fogginess". He was very pleased with his overall result. He was ready to take a new position at a high-tech start-up company and was very excited for his future. Two years on, he is still functioning at a very optimized level.

CHAPTER 22

What do we make of all this?

Taking a few steps back, it is amazing to think that just swallowing a few little pills would make such a big difference in the lives of so many people. It seems unlikely that a person suffering from constant symptoms, which invade every nook and cranny of life, can be so easily changed for the better. And yet, instead, so many patients report having been told by medical professionals that they would get so much better if only they would buckle down and try harder to pay attention. My response? "I must have missed that lecture." Seriously, though, it is clear that these professionals, while well-intentioned, likely do not fully understand Attention Deficit Disorder and how it can be approached and treated.

I emphasize to my patients that their symptoms are not a failure of their character. But even my patients are at first reluctant to believe that their lifelong "bad habits" and/or tendencies can really be changed. It is very confusing to learn that taking a medication can transform your life in a way that should only be attainable through a deep commitment to changing your behaviour and personality. I often tell my patients that if I didn't do this work all day long, I wouldn't believe it either.

The fact that the medical, psychiatric, and psychological professions have advanced so little in their understanding and treatment of ADD is reflective of this stuck-in-limbo state of affairs. To this day, most mental health professionals have both a very suspicious and, at the same time, moralizing tone in their approach to ADD. But this phenomenon is no different than anything that confronts and challenges society, forcing people to overcome their entrenched belief systems. Prejudice against people based on their "otherness"—whether it be racial or religious or gender-based—often sparks the reflex reaction to recoil in fear and maintain the status quo. It wasn't so long ago that my profession viewed homosexuality as a mental illness, for instance. That fact looks sadly wrongheaded now of course, but it was the prevailing belief system only a few decades ago.

What helps any of us overcome our "wrongheadedness"? Learning about issues, education, exposure to new and different ideas, becoming familiar with the "other". When it comes down to it, seeing another perspective is really what this book is about. Understanding the basis of the likely issues that underpin the causality in the case of the ADD patient. Having a treatment model that not only accounts for symptomatology but also provides a "feedback loop" that guides treatment direction going forward. That is what this book is about.

If I were asked what is the aim of the treatment protocol I have outlined, my answer might surprise a lot of readers. Certainly there are target symptoms that one expects to improve significantly. But my real aim with my patients is to enhance and maximize their freedom.

The fact is, almost all of my adult ADD patients are essentially "prisoners" trapped inside an inaccurate and fixed perspective of themselves. The way they know themselves is the way they have always been. They have their successes and failures like everyone, but their internal belief system is ultimately that they are damaged goods. They can't be normal and regular and effective. They just can't, they feel. And as they live their lives, they feel more and more certain that their self-concept, their understanding of their true self, is this diminished state of not being good enough.

And they are wrong. I don't say that to make my patients feel better. I say that to be accurate. They are wrong.

What the treatment protocol provides then is not just the opportunity for symptom reduction but also for the chance to operate and function in a manner consistent with the person's capacity, intellect, and intent—often for the first time in their life. That possibility is what lures people away from their fixed (and negative) belief system about themselves. Then, after a sustained period of observing how much better they are doing, they come to the realization that their former self-concept wasn't set in stone and they are able to finally entertain a new view of themselves. Not because the new story is better than the old story but because the new story is more accurate. It is this sharper sense of accuracy, this sense of no longer being resigned to this internally crippling belittled sense of self that provides the enhancement of personal freedom we all seek. And this is the reason I often say to my patients that they are getting a chance to meet themselves for the first time. Their true self.

Let me now move to a broader consideration of what we call Attention Deficit Disorder. One huge advantage I have had, at least from an overall perspective of ADD, is that I have treated people of all ages, not just children struggling with paying attention in the classroom, not just teenagers avoiding completing their assignments. I also treat adults who manifest very significant difficulties managing their lives in multiple areas. As adults, they have lived longer and are in a position where they are making their own decisions and seeing the consequences of their actions all the time.

My untreated yet-to-be-diagnosed adult ADD patients almost always have a history of problems in multiple areas. They often have trouble keeping their weight steady and frequently carry 20 extra pounds on their frame. At some point, they have had to regain control over one or more "vices"—alcohol, cigarette smoking, marijuana use, street drugs, and/or promiscuity. Almost all will have a sense that their mood control, including anxiety management, is weak and "all over the place". Many have had multiple failed efforts in relationships and marriage. Many have suffered bitter disappointments in college and university and/or in frequent job loss and career failure. They can be wildly inconsistent in parenting roles.

They also come with a shopping bag full of diagnoses. If you are an ADD person reading this book,

see how many of these words have been used by doctors to describe
you along the path you have thus far travelled:

- Depressed
- Bipolar
- Anxious
- Personality Disorder
- Oppositional/Defiant
- Borderline
- Substance Abuser
- Eating Disorder/Bulimia
- Narcissistic
- Obsessive-Compulsive

What is obvious in all of these domains is the common
thread of the central challenge of self-regulation. As stated earlier, I
have often felt that the term "Self-Regulation Deficiency Disorder"
(SRDD) would be a much more accurate and comprehensive
diagnostic term for ADD. Such a term would help to reposition the
broader understanding of the core issues that people face and would
de-emphasize the "attention" and "hyperactivity" aspects that I see as
just part of the many areas of dysregulation that ADD people
struggle with. This "SRDD" feature is richly on display in the
following two case examples.

CASE #1 – Caroline

Caroline was referred for consultation by her family doctor. A real estate agent in her early thirties, she noted, "I can't remember what I go into a room for." She felt very disorganized and noted "poor attention to detail" which is very important in her line of work. "I can't remember where things are and I have to go over things numerous times. My rational thought is not there." She also stated, "My procrastination is at an all-time high, even for the simplest tasks." She felt she was "good with people" but confessed that she frequently interrupted her clients when they were trying to speak with her.

Caroline smoked half a pack of cigarettes per day and had struggled in her late twenties with alcohol following the sudden accidental death of her fiancé. She had suffered with an eating disorder (bulimia) from the age of 13 into her early twenties. She had been assessed as having a learning disability when she was in elementary school. In her mid-teens, she was treated with Prozac and counselling for depression.

She dropped out of college early and floated through a series of jobs. Because she intuitively felt smarter than how she had done in school, and because of her personable ability with people, she decided to take the real estate sales agent course. She worked very hard and, when it came to examination time, she was able to get very high marks with the help of her brother's stimulant medication.

The other striking feature in her family history was the presence of alcoholism and depression on both sides of her family tree.

On examination, her mood was somewhat anxious, which she attributed to the acute stress she felt being constantly unprepared and easily flustered. She felt that her friends would describe her as a "bit flaky" with respect to making plans but would say she is a good friend. She was clearly intelligent, articulate, and despite her anxious strain, somewhat confident in her personal manner. She noted that as her income was commission-based, it was hugely important for her to be able to function at a higher level than she was. She wanted to have more control over her life and how she operated on a day-to-day basis. She subscribed to all of the 18 symptoms of the Adult Self-Report Scale for ADD.

Caroline clearly had ADD but she had never been diagnosed with it, never treated for it. Why? For all the reasons I have written about. She was nice and pretty. She was female, not male. All of the "noise" of her lack of close self-control—depressed mood, anxiety, eating disorders, alcohol use, not sticking with things, being too flighty— was just overlooked. But if someone along the way had said, "I think you have a self-regulation difficulty and, guess what, there's something that we can do about it," maybe that would have allowed her to more successfully navigate the tricky business of adolescence and young adulthood.

What ensued? Caroline came back for her education session and it resonated strongly for her, given her life experiences and frustrations. She was started on my treatment protocol with short-acting Dexedrine and returned one week later to report on this treatment regimen:

- 1 ½ tablets in the morning
- 1 tablet after lunch
- 1 tablet in the later afternoon

Caroline reported negligible side effects. She observed that she was definitely more productive with clearer thinking, less hyperness and feeling much more composed.

Her dosage was adjusted and tailored over the next 9 days to:

- 2 tablets in the morning
- 2 tablets after lunch
- 1 ½ tablets in the later afternoon

Caroline was manifestly changed—more focused and less fidgety. She also felt more motivated but noted that, although she was procrastinating less than she used to, it was "still there." She was responding so well that we decided to maintain her treatment and review her progress in three weeks. Seen at that time, my clinical notes read as follows:

- Procrastination issues minimal
- Feeling "really good"
- Work is amazing; so productive; more confident
- "I feel better about myself"

Again, it was determined she should stay the course and review two weeks further on.

By the next appointment, Caroline was able to discern that her procrastination issues were still more than they should be and that other aspects of her executive functioning, particularly prioritization and time management, could still be improved on. She had already exhibited an excellent Stage I response but that was still not giving her the full opportunity that she needed. We decided to start the Stage II protocol—Wellbutrin XL 150 mg every morning for the first week followed by Wellbutrin XL 300 mg in the second week, barring side effects.

Seen two weeks later, Caroline had her "neurotransmission" full engaged. "I just do. I don't sit around dwelling endlessly on the task. My mind is clear. I'm much more confident. And I'm not procrastinating." Caroline's nervous presentation was long gone. In its place was a more integrated and strikingly natural representation of her "true self".

The reasons for Caroline's transformation, though obvious to me, are debatable. Many well-intended people would object to my reliance (and Caroline's) on medication. Some would attribute her improvement to the personal experience of being cared for. Others would impute a response to my charisma (I wish). But what is indisputable is that Caroline was dramatically improved in the direction that was consistent with her intellect, her capacity, and her intentionality. And, ADD aside, she was vastly more able to self-regulate.

Let's let Caroline's description of her experience complete the consideration of her case before we turn to the second case that highlights the self-regulation issues.

CASE #1 – Caroline's Follow Up

"I have been working with Dr. Hoffer for about 3 months now and to

say my overall mindset and ability to function is at a "normal" level would be an understatement. When I first came to see Dr. Hoffer, I was sceptical. I had been passed back and forth between doctors throughout my life, so why would this be any different? If I knew then what I know now, I would have sought him out years ago.

At my first session, Dr. Hoffer bluntly said to me: You have a functioning disorder. He used the example of my glasses to describe how the medication would assist me in day-to-day life: The medication is much like your glasses, you or your eyes are not diseased, you do not have cataracts or anything like that, but you need glasses and the glasses help you to see more clearly. At this point, I was introduced to Stage 1 of the 2-Stage treatment.

I was first put on the Dextroampheta in a gradual dose over a week and a half period and really started to notice a difference in my day-to-day life. There were a few side effects of dry mouth, lack of appetite (you have to make sure you eat) and moments after taking the medication, my heart beat would get faster for a few minutes, but those side effects, aside from the lack of appetite, disappeared in a few days.

After that, I was more alert, focused, could pay attention to people without losing interest and blanking out in a matter of seconds like I had mostly done in the past. I got up in the morning and was able to start my day without hesitation. I would no longer linger in bed with the anxieties I would have about the tasks I knew I would struggle with or not complete. I started to have confidence in my decisions, my choices and myself. The need to over-analyze every task started to disappear, I was starting to feel like the me I knew I always was but never thought I could be. It was as if I had been living in the dark this whole time and someone slowly took a dimmer switch and turned on the light.

The light really brightened when Dr. Hoffer added the second aspect of my treatment, Wellbutrin. I had heard of this medication before to treat depression as a few family members had been prescribed this, but for me, it was for procrastination. In the past, the simplest tasks would be like climbing Mount Everest. I would overthink the task and then stress out about it, then get anxiety about the stress, which then would lead me to shutting down and if I didn't think about it then it didn't exist. Procrastinating was as common as breathing to me on a day-to-day basis.

Much like the first introduction to the Dexedrine, the Wellbutrin took a few days to notice a change in my day-to-day life. I almost missed the change because I stopped overthinking tasks or decisions; I would just do and complete. If I knew I needed to do something, I did it. Simple, right? Never for me. I started preparing myself for the next day to make sure I was ready. I have become organized, paying attention to detail, taking time to go through things to understand fully what is being asked of me. The dimmer light turned to its fullest brightness.

These medications have changed my life in the best way possible. I have suffered from eating disorders, depression, lack of self confidence, all due to my lack of being able to function and perform as good as the next person. I was constantly comparing myself and asking myself, what is wrong with me? Today, after just under three months of being on these medications, I am not a new me but I am the me I always knew I could be. I am confident, happy with myself, I smile more, I am active, articulate and more driven. I have never been more content in my life. It is visible in my work, my relationships and on my face. For the first time in my life, I am excited about what is next and what the future will bring for me and not because of a foreign entity but because I will be the one getting me there."

CASE #2 — Rebecca

Rebecca, who was 10 years younger than Caroline, was alerted to the possibility that she may have Attention Deficit Disorder symptoms by her psychotherapist. After speaking with a few medical sources, she asked her family doctor to request a referral to see me.

Rebecca was full of charm and personality. Vivacious and quick witted, intelligent and personable, she had graduated from university and had entered the business world as a middle management recruiter/headhunter. She arrived at my office with this written history:

"I am not exactly sure where to start or how to sum up the issues I've had over the years. I first remember the problems starting when I was maybe 12 or 13, when I was starting to misbehave and disobey my parents. By 14 or 15, I was very sexually active. I would do kind of outrageous stuff like sleep with two guys in one night or sneak out of my aunt's house and take her car and go see some guy. I took $20 bills from my parents' wallets and crashed their vehicle. I used the fact that I did well in school as leverage to not get in trouble. I ended up screwing up a lot of friendships and causing huge fights in my household just because I was so set on doing what I wanted and totally disregarded what I was asked to do.

I was very active. I danced and taught dance classes in the community and was on student council and did very well in school until the end of high school. I was a top student and well liked. I guess this is why no one worried too much. I *got into McGill and moved to Montreal, and my behaviour just continued. I partied more than most people at school. I always had to be the centre of attention, which got me into trouble or embarrassing situations. I drink often until I black out. I use cocaine, which comes and goes in phases. I have had times where I use a lot, 4 times a week, and times now where it's pretty rarely. I am completely incapable of budgeting or not overspending. I have over $50,000 in student debt, and my parents have repeatedly bailed me out. To this day, I run my bank account dry every week. I ignore my bills.*

I didn't do that great in university, but I graduated. High school was really easy because there wasn't much competition and I remember never having to try very hard. I do well at work but I can never seem to get ahead or on top of what my goals are. I am disorganized and bad with deadlines. I feel like I am always falling short of my potential and my reckless and irresponsible behaviour holds me back. I screw up the relationships I've been in because I cheat or do stupid stuff.

Most of my friends and people in my life really love me and think of me as this crazy, fun loving, free spirited girl. I've always just thought I have a really wild big excited personality, but I am kind of coming to terms with my problems. My family finally pushed me to get some help after my psychotherapist, Dr. Eliana Cohen, told me she thinks all of this stuff is because I have ADHD."

I took her history. Rebecca had the classic "Hofferian" duality of ADD symptoms—difficulty sustaining attention if not interested coupled with huge procrastination issues. She told me, "I can't get a hold of my life. I can't stop doing the things that cause me problems." She couldn't get around to getting her laundry done or paying her bills. She undermined her chances for promotion by not completing a relatively simple Excel spreadsheet assignment. She felt her impulse control was weak. "I do whatever I want to do when I can do it." She felt she lacked a pause button. She constantly finished other people's sentences. Alcohol use verged on the problematic.

Rebecca then went through my usual treatment protocol. First, we had an education session. Rebecca decided to initiate treatment so we started on the Stage I stimulant. She was dramatically improved within the first two weeks. "I'm able to sit and work for two hours without going to the bathroom or getting a snack." She felt much more confidant.

Her dose was tailored. Seen two weeks later, she was still doing much better. Seen two weeks after that, it was clear that she still required strengthening of her Stage II/executive function/procrastination issues. Wellbutrin XL was initiated with 150 mg tablets. Eleven days later, she was already "more aware of the decision-making process." She was more motivated at work and had cleared her apartment. Since she is diminutive in size, we decided not to increase the Wellbutrin dose. Seen three weeks later, Rebecca reported that she was doing great, feeling very organized. She had been promoted at work and felt much more in control of herself.

Like Caroline, Rebecca was no longer plagued with self doubt and negative self-talk. Properly treated, she was finally feeling like herself. Next up: Her perspective on her life transformation following ADD treatment.

CASE #2 – Rebecca's Follow Up

"My name is Rebecca and I am 23 years old. I saw Dr. Hoffer for the first time 10 weeks ago. That's not very long, and you might not even believe this story and the drastic differences, but it's all true. It's hard to explain exactly what's happened but I'll do my best. I haven't changed at all, yet everything about what I do is different. The change is subtle, but the impact is more than you can understand.

What tipped my parents over the edge after years of exasperation with my behaviour was that I got completely blackout drunk at a family function. For the first time, they paid for me to see a therapist. I babbled and told stories for just two sessions, and she identified the problem. Randomly and luckily, as many things seem to happen in my life, I had a good friend in university whose Dad I knew to be a psychiatrist specializing in adult ADHD. I cold called him and he agreed to see me.

When I first went to see Dr. Hoffer, he asked me to write 3 - 4 paragraphs of what brought me there. The paragraphs highlighted the behaviours I had exhibited since my early teens. These behaviours ranged between mischievous to delinquent to endearing to scary. Excessive spending, excessive drinking and drug use, extreme promiscuity, and generally a complete disregard for consequences in order to enjoy myself in the moment and live my life the way I wanted to. The contrast to this was that I was loved by family and friends and was outgoing, charming, and quite successful academically. I was smart and savvy and charismatic and it appears no one could stay mad at me for long. If you had asked me to describe myself six months ago, I would have done so with self-affection. Complex, fervent, spiraling beautiful mess.

But it was the truth of it that would hit me like a bag of bricks when I'd run out of money and my power would go out because I'd spent the money that was meant for hydro at the bar. And I'd have breakdowns and feel really lost and incapable of… I'm not even sure—I just felt incapable. I'd feel confused about why I couldn't go out and drink moderately. I'd feel confused about why repeatedly I would wind up at home and not have any clue how I got there, or worse, in someone's backyard so disoriented that they called the cops to drive me home. I'd feel confused about why I couldn't get my damn alarm to wake me up and I'd be late for work again.

Before I knew about any of this, I started writing a little story that I thought would maybe be a chapter of a book I'd write someday. I compared myself to Scarlett O'Hara, a tragic hero who loved herself and knew that she was special. In a twisted way, she loved herself because she continually messed shit up for herself due to her impulses. It was a part of her identity, but the end of the book is sad.

So, I went to see Dr. Hoffer because I'd been told I had ADHD and then the Wikipedia page sounded a whole lot like me. I was excited to have an answer—but extremely nervous to change, and to lose parts of me that had become my identity.

I sat down to see him and we chatted a bit. He told me in a teasing and kind way that I was boring him because my case was so clean cut. And he told me that he knew he could help me and that he knew exactly what was going to happen to me if I followed his treatment.

He explained the neuroscience behind ADHD. The part about the outer cortex and concentration didn't worry me. I had taken stimulants in university to study and they had made me feel like a superhuman who was organized, on the ball, and 10 times more powerful than my normal self. Then he

240

started to talk about Stage II. This is the part about executive functioning, and for this, he prescribes Wellbutrin, which is generally considered to be an antidepressant, and this part worried me.

I was worried that I would start taking this drug and that I would start to lose the wild parts of me that I understood as my personality. My friends knew me as crazy wild fun Rebecca. I knew myself this way too. I'd accepted the wildness and taught myself to love it so I was scared for a drug to take that away. I remember asking about this in my first meeting with Dr. Hoffer, and just as he predicted every single other thing that's happened, he told me that I wouldn't lose those parts, but be able to control them and choose them and tame them if I want to.

I started treatment (working up to just over 20 mg of Dexedrine per day). Immediately, I saw differences in my work life. I was more focused and productive and I got promoted about one month later. I felt alert and busy and like I could accomplish whatever was put in front of me, when previously I showed this face, but often felt overwhelmed and demotivated on the inside.

One month in, I started taking the Wellbutrin. After just two weeks, some very, very interesting things started to happen. I was shopping with my closest friend who I hadn't seen in several months. I tried on and picked out a black sleeveless blouse for work. It was somewhere in the $60 range on the tag which seemed reasonable. When the cashier rang it up, it came out just over $80. I stood at the cash and I'm sure the thought process and turmoil of "Do I buy it or not?" was plainly written on my face. After a few screwed facial expressions, I apologetically blurted out to the cashier that I couldn't justify spending 80 bucks on a black tank top, and that I was sorry she rang it up but I wasn't going to purchase it. Jenny, my friend and a psychology major, quietly watched this happen.

She then told me that she couldn't believe what she had just seen. She had never seen me act so rationally or consequentially and was thrilled to have witnessed the changes that were happening in my life.

I've got a pause button now. Dr. Hoffer described it as a pause button when I first went to see him. It's a pause button that people with ADHD don't naturally have. Now I have this ability to make a choice in the moment. I can honestly tell you I've never experienced this before six weeks ago. Sure, in the past, I knew there was a choice available to me, but it didn't matter. I was going to choose what felt good at the time, every single time, despite the consequences.

The coolest part about all of this is that I can still choose to do what feels good in the moment if I want to. I have no plans of being "square" or "boring" or not the centre of attention for that matter. But now, a real choice in my actions is available to me, where I can understand and weigh the consequences of either avenue. I feel in control. I feel like myself, and my personality is just as vibrant as it's ever been, but I haven't blacked out from drinking once since starting the second course of treatment. I can think, "I should probably wait 30 minutes before I have another drink. That's a good idea."

I feel different, and I feel better, and I feel like I'm on a path where I am moving forward all the time, rather than zig-zagging and crisscrossing and not really knowing where I was going.

I am so grateful to my parents, and my friends, and to the therapist who figured it out when no one else saw it, and to Dr. Hoffer for making my life totally different but keeping me as the same person. Before, I called myself a complex, fervent, spiraling beautiful mess. And I'll always love this person that I was and she'll always be a part of me. Now however, the words I choose to describe how I feel about myself are a complex, passionate, positive, capable, confident, and enthusiastic young lady. If you compare the two, some of the words would probably show up beside each other in a thesaurus. The differences are subtle on the outside, but on the inside, they are allowing me to be my best self."

CHAPTER 23

How can you live your best life?

It is always interesting to read about people's life circumstances and follow how they find their way. It is even more interesting when there is a psychiatric aspect to our own personal search for a deeper understanding of the human condition, what makes us tick, what makes us who we are. Once we delve into a new subject and start learning, it's easy to become impressed by change, especially when—as illustrated by the patient cases presented here—the outcomes are so positive.

Shortly after I started writing this book, I was approached by the highly regarded documentary filmmaker Michael McNamara to participate in a film about Adult Attention Deficit Disorder. He and I met a few times and I was impressed by his award-winning career of thoughtfully constructed and fair-minded documentary work and his genuine interest in the subject matter. But I was leery of media involvement in the case of Attention Deficit Disorder. Doctors hardly understand this area and media, who tend to share that "drugs are bad and doctors who prescribe are worse" perspective, often manipulate stories to serve a misinformed belief system. I made it clear to Mr. McNamara that if he was going to do the usual "Does ADD exist?" documentary with one doctor pontificating in front of a large bookcase that ADD is a figment of pharmaceutical companies' imagination created for the evil purpose of conning the general public into buying their wares while I appear on the other side of the screen insisting that I treat ADD all day long, then count me out. I told him he would have no problem finding many doctors who would be excited just to be on television but that I was not one of them.

Now, if, on the other hand, he could create a far more useful documentary, one which would challenge the status quo and elevate the discourse about ADD in the field of medicine, I would definitely consider being involved. Our intentions aligned, I did go on to participate in this film, along with Robert Pal, an outstanding ADD coach with whom I often collaborate in the treatment of people with ADD, as well as a number of patients that I would be seeing. The documentary film is scheduled to air in Spring 2017 on The Nature of Things on CBC (Canadian Broadcasting Corporation) and then will be available for watching online.

Now, it would have been relatively easy to simply "cherry pick" patients who had successful treatment outcomes, both for this book and for the documentary film. Everyone who treats Attention Deficit Disorder has had some success, particularly for the minority of ADD patients who respond well to just one medication. That is why medical clinicians do not and should not rely on anecdotal reports of "one-offs"—single cases that had great outcomes with an innovative treatment approach.

The real therapeutic value comes when there is a defined treatment protocol based on a well worked-through treatment model. At my insistence, and in order to maintain the integrity of the process, patients were chosen as I started their assessment and treatment, as opposed to pre-selecting only the "success stories". As I told Mr. McNamara, I am confident in the approach that I use every day in my clinical practice and therefore I had no need to bias the outcome.

Close to 20 years ago, I wrote the first few chapters of a book somewhat similar, though not as conceptually advanced, as this one. I sent it off to a serious literary agent in New York City. He thought it was pretty good, with new and important thinking that deserved to be published. He presented it to an important publishing house and the manuscript quickly moved up the chain of command to the person who decided yes or no. The agent relayed the sad story of what happened next. The publishing executive went to the Amazon website, which was then used primarily for selling books, and typed in "ADD". He got back 400 titles in his search. He called the agent back and declined the book on the basis that he felt he couldn't make a business case for publishing the 401st book on the subject. Despite his acknowledgement that he felt what I was writing was important, even valuable, he just didn't consider it publishable.

Now normally, I wouldn't have given up with just one

rejection. But as I found myself uncharacteristically put off by the lunacy of that process, I set aside the book project and got on with the business of life. My children were young then and I couldn't justify the time spent away from my family. I would get back to it one day, I promised myself. Really, I would.

Months passed. Years passed. Generations of people with ADD grew up—with inadequate or even no treatment. So many lives were unfulfilled. As for me, I was doing my own work with my own patients. Really, what more could I do?

A couple of years ago, an adult ADD patient of mine whom I had treated for several years was in my office for a check-up appointment. His life had been turned around some eight years prior and over time, he frequently mentioned how grateful he was that his life had taken a turn in a vastly more successful direction. Now and again, he would ask if I was planning to write a book so I could share my treatment approach with others, so more people could benefit from ADD treatment the way he had. I would answer in a half-hearted way with "I'm planning to get around to it when I can find the time," or I'd get defensive and say, "I give frequent talks to other doctors." This time, however, he tackled the issue straight on: "You are always going to be busy. But there are legions of people out there who, like me, are searching all the time to find a doctor who has any clue about this. Writing a book to share it more widely isn't something you should get around to; it is moral imperative."

This ADD patient, this man whose life had been transformed, was not only very eloquent, he was right. I was proud of what I was accomplishing in my clinical practice and I have always been generous in sharing my protocols with other clinicians. But entire generations of people, from young to old, are suffering with a terrible functional problem that the overwhelming proportion of the mental health treatment world still approaches, if at all, with an understanding that stopped advancing in the 1970's.

But there is a significant consideration that needs to be stated. Many doctors would point out that, moral imperative aside, what I have written about in this book, well-intended as it may be, has not been put through a formal clinical research trial. They may state that while the clinical case examples are impressive, they remain entertaining anecdotal case reports until they are put through properly constructed double blind studies.

They are right. And wrong. Permit me to explain.

It would be a very neat and orderly world if everything that we do in medicine could be subjected to clinical trials and research studies. But it is not so neat, especially in the world of psychiatry, where so much of what is done doesn't easily lend itself to physical world measurements, such as blood tests and MRI scans. In fact, the kind of work that I am describing, in which medications are tailored to the individual clinical response and many patients are on two or more medications at once, does not easily lend itself to research design. Moreover, the time and cost to do so would be significant and prohibitive.

Also, we can't discount the unique set of experiences that has propelled my work in the area of Attention Deficit Disorder. These experiences can and will never be replicated. Just because the resulting theory is the product of many decades of clinical work, as opposed to more typical research, doesn't make it less valid. In fact, my whole purpose in writing of this book was to provide a constructive, working framework that has been tested in order to create a basis of dialogue for moving forward in a stale and complacent area of psychiatry.

We've all heard the saying "If I had a nickel for every time I heard (fill in the blank), I'd be rich". For me, it would be some variation of these phrases: "I wish I had been treated ten years ago because everything would have been so much different." "I wouldn't have screwed up my life. I would have finished school. I wouldn't have thought I was stupid all those years." "I would have been able to be a better spouse/father/friend." The literal carnage that unrecognized ADD, or ADD that is only partially treated, visits upon a person's life and that of their loved ones can be devastating. And the saddest part is that it is so avoidable.

The other phase that I hear so often is "Why didn't the clinicians I saw before tell me about this?" Or "Why didn't they try harder?" I constantly explain to patients that not everybody knows enough about treating ADD and too many people aren't confident about it.

Of course, some people will only want to address this problem two or three decades from now, when the few studies that are finally done in the area have been widely disseminated. But you are likely reading this book because you don't want to wait 20 or 30 more years to address the vast gulf between where you are and where you intuitively know you can and should be. And you don't have to. Anyone who is touched by Attention Deficit Disorder can read this book. They can share it with their loved ones. They can have their doctors and therapists read it. They can search for a willing ear. They can try to find a solution because they will finally have a way forward and a roadmap to follow. Now you know that if you were losing hope, or you if you haven't felt hope before, you don't have to give up.

We all know about the unfortunate lingering stigma that is associated with mental illness. But keep in mind one of the major tenets of this book, which is that ADD is not an illness but a disorder of self-regulatory function. Still, the subject of mental illness remains an obstacle in ADD cases, and not only with respect to the general public but also inside the helping profession.

A perfect example of this stigma was illustrated in the documentary on adult ADD that I referenced earlier. I referred to two patients that I had just assessed as classic Stage I/Stage II patients. One was a social worker on the verge of losing her job. The other was a medical student struggling to complete his studies. Both were in their thirties. Both ended up having transformational clinical responses. Both ended up deciding against sharing their stories on film because they both feared that doing so could potentially harm their professional careers. Even though both were hugely grateful and both worked in helping professions and both well understood how important their stories would be to thousands of others, they could not overcome their own personal concerns. One patient went on to share her story here instead.

"I am the fourth child in a family of six children, raised in a two-parent household. My parents are originally from West Africa, Ghana, and our family migrated to Canada when I was three. Culturally, academics was the focus and stated sole purpose of our lives as children. My parents enrolled us in every extracurricular lesson possible and had high expectations from us, mainly from our report cards.

Sadly, I was a constant disappointment in that area. Although dutiful and obedient, I was never able to master the art of academics. Middle and secondary school teachers characterized me as a 'well intentioned, disorganized mess.' I tried hard but seemed to never get it right. My parents interpreted my lack of accomplishment as a deliberate act of sabotage against their dreams of creating academic achievers. Thus, our relationship became tainted and I, unlike my siblings, was routinely made the butt of many hurtful jokes. It was only when my sixth grade teacher, Mr. B, in a difficult parent teacher conference, alluded to my parents that I might have a learning disorder, that I thought maybe it wasn't me but my challenges that caused my parents such pain. As quickly as it was mentioned, the idea was dismissed and attributed to a school system that labels black students and sees them 'deficient and stupid.'

My parents divorced when I was in high school, we siblings were divided, and I with my younger sisters were sent to live with my mother. No longer in a high pressured environment and managing to build some self confidence, my focus became to prove my disparagers wrong, that I was capable for success. Whether it took me five hours to complete a 1-page assignment or that I had to study for a quiz months in advance, I did it, with favorable results. However, with each

success came a growing sense of panic that it all wasn't sustainable, and that
eventually I would be found out. School president, affable, accomplished, the
exterior shell I presented to the world would be shattered if some little piece of my
well-crafted world came loose.

Here enters caffeine. A friend of mine, noticing my need for fuel,
suggested that I drink coffee. This was well before the Starbucks or Tim Hortons
heyday. Caffeine helped me survive; however, by grade 13, I was burnt out and
petrified. Accepted to the University of Toronto, I was fearful about whether I
could really make it in a much bigger pond, with heavier demands. My
apprehension was well founded, because university was a mess, I switched majors
five times and completed my Bachelor's degree in six and a half years. A
sympathetic professor once said this about me, "... you present so well." Words
were hurled like knives, by well-intentioned friends, family members and partners:
"Why can't you pull yourself together?" "You need to find your balance."

I simply couldn't keep up. I was overwhelmed by it all. The pressure of
achievement caused my stress levels to explode as I imploded. I simply gave up. I
didn't understand why I couldn't cope, why I would sit in front of a computer for
literally days and would produce a paragraph, my mind unable to focus. I was
constantly panicked and depleted. When I did graduate, I took a year off and did
some introspection. A friend of mine who I opened up to about my struggles gave
me the book 'Scattered Minds' by Gabor Mate. I found myself within the pages of
his book and attempted to put his advice to good use, and for a period of time,
things were clearer. I felt I now knew who the enemy was and it wasn't me. I
completed my Master's degree in two albeit not one year, but I did not battle
feelings of self loathing that had plagued me during my Bachelor's. During this
time, I read a ton of self-help material, did manualized CBT, developed lists, used

time management strategies, practiced mindfulness, and learned to say no.

I thought I had it in the bag, that I was well on my way, new relationship, great job. Within eight months, I had lost it all, my partner left, telling me he couldn't live in the chaos, that I was life sucking. One employer kindly suggested that I was perhaps not cut out for this line of work and suggested a less demanding profession. Now, three jobs later, sitting at my boss' desk waiting for the inevitable chastisement, she tells me that she values me and thinks I need help, that similar to me, she lives with impulsivity and distraction. I am again hopeful.

With the guidance of my employer, a dash of providence and spurred by the possibility of better, I successfully booked my first appointment with Dr. Mayer Hoffer. I approached the meeting with great skepticism but left just enough room for 'something'. Thankfully, I got more than expected. In two simple sentences, my conscience was cleared, I was absolved, I wasn't a failure, I wasn't incompetent, I had a functional disorder, my brain wasn't like others, and moreover, it didn't have to stay that way, it could change and I could be the girl who seemed so far out of reach, the true me.

Like a new convert, eager for redemption but wary of being misled, I approached each meeting cautiously. Aware of my desperation and vulnerability, I received factual information, I learned of dopamine, of synapses and neurotransmitters, I received acknowledgement, encouragement, hope and then a little orange triangular pill that turned my world upside down, right side up. Pure sorcery, magic, normal, for the first time in a long time I was able to function, function at work, at home, with friends, life became manageable, the possibilities grew. It took some adjustment and a couple of additions to the chemical brew, and then I arrived at normal. It took me some 30 plus years to get there, but I arrived.

I admit there were still challenges, the foremost being my lurking disbelief that my salve lay in a pharmacological intervention, a pill, not me, myself and sheer perseverance and grit. Self doubt, dare I say shame, crept up. I chastised myself with familiar words, 'western medication is bad,' 'taking medication is like giving up on you,' 'you want everything easy.'

My feelings of shame and doubt were also entangled and complicated by my need to both protect and desire not to reinforce stigmatizing, and negative characterizations of inaptitude, and 'unintelligence' often associated with black persons. I was at odds with myself, on the one hand thankful for the clarity that my diagnosis provided, but wary of the tainted implications that having an 'Attention Deficit Disorder' had in shaping my identity as an individual, as a racialized person and as a member of my family.

In conversations outside and in the safe space of Dr. Hoffer's office, I have been able to slowly come to terms with what it means to have a learning disorder. In addressing these difficult questions of 'identity' and 'ability', I have been challenged to get real with myself and have come to see this little pill as the missing piece of a puzzle that I had been constructing through grit and perseverance that completed what was already there.

Now almost a year into my treatment, what has changed? Everything, albeit in varying degrees. I am gainfully and happily employed. In my relationships with others, I have crawled from a place of shame-driven cynicism to cautious skepticism. I have not shared my diagnosis and treatment with my family because I believe they will not understand. Things still fall apart, to-do lists still litter the bottom of my purse, and I have yet to perfect the art of arriving on time or being socially well adjusted.

Most glaringly different is who and how I define and conceptualize myself to be. I no longer see myself as full of fault and deficiency. I now see myself as able, and surprisingly even better than able, dare I say accomplished. For now, and for me, this is more than enough, it's all I ever wanted, a chance at something more than I had.

Standing where I am now, filled with optimism and hunger for life, it is hard for me to connect with the girl from my past. That girl was worn down, frantic and tired. She seemed to always be on the brim of achieving excellence, but never getting there. She seemed to be always chasing possibility and possibility always evaded her. At times, I get angry and question why it took me so long to get help. Why so much had to be lost, why was I so afraid? These days, gratitude and understanding fill that space and I imagine a little girl similar to me, sitting quietly with her pain and self loathing and I hope that things will be easier…better, I am very hopeful of all the possibilities that could be made into reality."

As wonderful as the outcome can be for you, there is still a stigma associated with Attention Deficit Disorder, and it has to be recognized in order to be dealt with. Don't let this obstacle discourage you. Nobody ever said that getting the right help was going to be easy. Do not give up.

There are even more reasons to persevere. One reason, a big and important one, is that you may have children or you may plan to have a family one day, and there is a high probability that one or more of your children may have ADD as well. Count on it. You will want to know that they too can have happy and successful and fulfilling lives. So it's your job to lead the way by learning about

Attention Deficit Disorder and what can be done about it.

The degree of clinical improvement that can be achieved with children and teenagers is just as pronounced as it can be in adults. There is some irony that this book is primarily devoted to the consideration of ADD in adults. As I said, I plan to write a follow-up book about the treatment of ADD in children and teenagers. Interestingly, the books will come out in the opposite order of how my clinical experience developed. But in the end, it doesn't matter what age you are. No person with ADD has to be consigned to their fate. All ADD sufferers of all ages can have the lives they want; so can their children; so can their families.

The result of treatment model based clinical decision-making, as I have outlined, can "change the game" when it comes to Attention Deficit Disorder. But I am serious when I joke with patients that my treatment results are great but that the "optics" of what I do suck. There is no denying the long hard-fought battle I have endured in my clinical work as a psychiatrist specialist to get to the point where the clucking skeptics have finally started their orderly retreat. (The more shameless ones now claim that they were leading lights in recognizing the importance of ADD symptoms all along). Regardless, if we are consumed by optics, by political correctness, by the appearance of how we imagine things "should be", then the treatment protocols I have outlined here would never have been considered. And that would be a shame—because the results are clinically proven and they are not just good, and not just great. They are transformational.

As I said earlier in the book, if you are satisfied with the status quo, with using the same treatment approach for Attention Deficit Disorder that has existed unchanged for the past 40-50 years, then so be it. But I suspect you aren't so satisfied. And you want to do better in your own life, or in the life of your children, or you want to do better for your patients because too many people with ADD are suffering every day. Well, not anymore. Now you have a path forward, with built-in checks and balances along the way. Your life is about to change as soon as you take that step. Hope is here.

www.ingramcontent.com/pod-product-compliance
Lightning Source LLC
Chambersburg PA
CBHW051635170526
45167CB00001B/200